SELF MANAGE AND REVERSE YOUR DIABETES

By

Dr. GEETA SUNDAR-MD

Become
Shakespeare
.com

First published in 2016 by
BecomeShakespeare.com

Wordit Content Design & Editing Services Pvt Ltd
Quest Offices, C38/39, Parinee Crescenzo Building,
Bandra Kurla Complex, Bandra East,
Mumbai 400 051, India
T: +91 8080226699

ISBN 978-93-52017-08-9

Acknowldgement

My heartfelt and sincere thanks to the eminent Physician,. DR. YOGESH CHAWLA MD. DM. (GASTRO) FAMS, DIRECTOR, PROFESSOR AND HEAD DEPARMENT OF HEPATOLOGY, POST GRADUATE INSTITUTE OF MEDICAL EDUCATION AND RESEARCH, (PGI) CHANDIGARH -INDIA for finding time from his busy schedule to go through the manuscript and write a foreword.

And to my erudite class fellow—DR. ALOK DUBEY MBBS JABALPUR, M.D PAEDIATRICS AFMC PUNE, M. PHIL (HEALTH & HOSPITAL SYSTEMS MANAGEMENT) BITS PILANI for his meticulous editing and constructive criticism that helped to a great extent in bringing the manuscript to its final shape.

Foreword

स्नातकोत्तर चिकित्सा शिक्षा एवं अनुसंधान संस्थान, चण्डीगढ़ - 160 012 (भारत)
POSTGRADUATE INSTITUTE OF MEDICAL EDUCATION AND RESEARCH, CHANDIGARH - 160 012 (INDIA)

दूरभाष /Phone : (Off.) 0172-2748383, 2765556 , फैक्स / Fax: 01-172-2744401, 2745076
ई-मेल / E-mail: dpgi@pgimer.ccu.in वेबसाइट / Website http://pgimer.nic.in, nfr.@pgimer.gov.in

Dr. Yogesh Chawla
M D., D.N (GASTRO), F A M S
DIRECTOR
Professor & Head
Department of Hepatology

डॉ. योगेश चावला
एम.डी., डी.एम (गैस्ट्रो), एफ.ए.एम.एस
निदेशक
प्राचार्य एवं अध्यक्ष
यकृत रोग विभाग

संख्या / No. DPGI-7/8/1940
दिनांक / Date 18/8/15

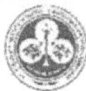

Diabetes is a global epidemic and there is a huge increase in the number of patients all over the world. While Diabetes has a strong genetic linkage, wrong lifestyle certainly adds to its incidence.

The book titled—'*Self manage and reverse your Diabetes*' by Dr. Geeta Sundar, demystifies all aspects of the disease including 'what is Diabetes', why some of us get afflicted, how it can be controlled and the respective roles of the doctor and patient. Is Diabetes a disease of Pancreas, Liver, Fat tissues, Muscles, or a problem primarily of the vascular system? In fact it is all of these as clearly brought out in the book.

I appreciate the narrative form taken by Dr. Geeta Sundar in explaining the functioning of Pancreas, Liver, and other organs with respect to Diabetes. The author very lucidly and successfully guides the reader on how to self manage his condition under the guidance of his doctor and how to work towards reversing it. She rightly points out that as of today Diabetes is not curable, but certainly one can try to reverse it.

The book is very comprehensive; covering all aspects of the disease including the complications arising out of Diabetes and their management. I am sure it will go a long way in assisting the patient with Diabetes in leading a normal life, help him to join the mainstream and reduce the treatment burden on society.

My heartiest congratulations to Dr. Geeta Sundar on bringing out such an informative and useful book. She has explained the science behind Diabetes and it's treatment in a simple language that can be understood by all. It has struck the right balance in being a 'must read book' for all patients suffering from Diabetes and doctors involved in treating it in a cost effective manner.

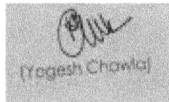

(Yogesh Chawla)

DR. YOGESH CHAWLA MD. DM. (GASTRO) FAMS

DIRECTOR PROFESSOR AND HEAD DEPARMENT OF HEPATOLOGY

POST GRADUATE INSTITUTE OF MEDICAL EDUCATION AND RESEARCH, CHANDIGARH – INDIA

Contents

PART-IV — PREVENTION AND REVERSAL

Introduction

Magnitude of the problem—why you need to understand self-management

Diabetes is a global epidemic and there is a huge increase in the number of patients all over the world. As per global projections by International Diabetes Federation (IDF), the number of diabetic patients in the world has risen sharply in recent years. While in 1985, 30 million people had diabetes worldwide; the number rose to 150 million in 2000, 285 million in 2010 and is estimated to be 435 million - 7.8% of the adult world population by 2030 resulting in direct medical costs of $376 billion ($116 billion in the United States). By 2030, the global incidence is projected to rise to 9.9 percent, partly because of the rising obesity rate, with costs reaching $490 billion.

In 2012, India had the highest number of diabetics in the world. By next year, the country will be home to 50.8 million diabetics, making it the world's unchallenged diabetes capital. And the number is expected to go up to 87 million – 8.4% of the country's adult population – Or to give a more scary perspective –

by 2030, every second Indian over the age of 50 will be a Diabetic

Considering this huge number of cases, doctors may not be able to spend enough time educating you about your disease. But you need to be trained scientifically so you can assume maximum responsibility for your own care. You should become well equipped to take decisions on a daily basis that will positively alter the course of your disease. Why is knowledge of self-management so important? Let me give you an example to prove my point. One of my patients (SD) was on insulin and was *fully trained in management of his disease*. He was returning from work on his company bus one day, when he felt uneasy. He calmly took out his glucometer, and tested his sugar—which was only 48mg%. His friend called me but said my patient knew what he had to do. Helped by his colleagues, SD quickly ate a packet of glucose biscuits and chocolates that he always carried and half an hour later still on the bus, felt well enough to call me himself saying his blood sugar was now 80mg%. I told him not to worry and to ask someone to receive him at his stop and take him home in a vehicle. On reaching home he should eat a banana and then some food. He was also instructed not to take his evening dose of insulin. He did as he was told, checked his blood glucose twice and when it came to 140mg% went off to sleep peacefully and came to see me next day. I was able to stabilise him in two days while he continued to go to work. This same patient if he had not been properly educated, would have panicked, been admitted and out of work for at least a week. He might also have gone into coma and become serious. That is the importance of being trained in self management. One must understand that blood glucose can change from day to day and hour to hour especially in those on insulin like in this patient of mine, and decisions for change in dose of medicine may have to be made frequently and quickly. For this it may not be possible for you to physically go to your doctor every time or for the doctor to give an immediate appointment. If you are fully trained, and able to monitor blood glucose, changes can quickly be made by contacting your doctor by — SMS/phone call/ or mail.

To self-manage your Diabetes; you have to first understand — what is diabetes, why blood sugar needs to be controlled, the need for Life style modification and how to go about it, self examination, self monitoring, recognizing complications, importance of regular checkups, maintaining a tracker, and setting self-goals. Once you become a *partner* in the management of your Diabetes, outcome and compliance will improve greatly and chances of complications will reduce. Another important thing to understand is that — *there are bound to be setbacks during the course of the disease,* but you should remain positive and overcome them. Blood sugar is affected by what you eat, how much or how little you exercise, whether you get enough sleep, how stressed you are, among other factors. So fluctuations *will* occur and you must respond to them as quickly as possible before they get out of hand.

By the time you finish reading this book, I hope you will have learnt to manage about 60% of your Diabetes on your own, leaving the remaining 40% comprising monitoring and advising medication, to your doctor.

You will find that I have repeated a few things several times — this is to re-enforce this information so that you remember it. Once you have reached this stage, you can go on to the next step — YES! Attempt to reverse your Diabetes, which I will tell you about at the end of the book. *Let me caution you — reversal is not cure. Reversal is going backwards, and trying to undo the whole process by which you got Diabetes.* But don't jump the gun! You cannot attempt reversal, without a thorough understanding of Diabetes. So let me take it step by step —

PART I

UNDERSTANDING DIABETES

Chapter 1

WHAT IS DIABETES? HOW DOES IT OCCUR?

Diabetes is called 'Madhumeha' in Sanskrit, which literally means sweet urine.

It is a disease of "starvation amidst plenty" because although the blood is rich in sugar, this cannot be utilized by the body. Many of you know that insulin is required by the body for utilizing the sugar obtained from food and is secreted by Beta or Islet cells in the Pancreas — a leaf shaped organ in the abdomen that lies inside the loop of the first part of the intestines called 'duodenum'. Its secretions are insulin, and many digestive enzymes that digest fat, carbohydrates and proteins.

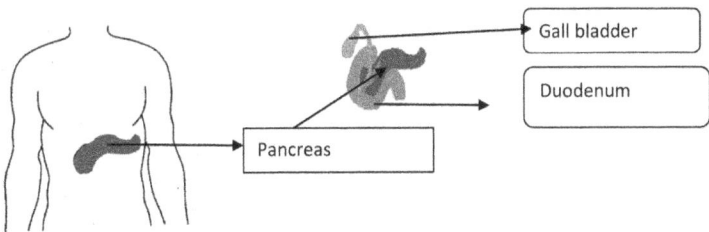

Insulin is like a key that opens the lock for glucose to enter the cells and be utilized to produce energy

Without insulin therefore, glucose cannot enter the cells. It keeps accumulating in the blood and results in a disease we all know as diabetes.

Pancreas also secretes 'glucagon', which acts opposite to insulin, that is, it raises blood glucose when it becomes low.

Pancreas additionally secretes digestive juices. Digestive juices besides helping in digestion of carbohydrates, fats, and proteins, are highly alkaline and neutralize the acidic contents that come from the stomach into the duodenum.

Diabetes occurs due to lack of insulin–Type I Diabetes or to a defect in the action of insulin — Type-II Diabetes. The first is easy to understand because if there is no insulin, sugar cannot be utilized by the body. But in the second type of diabetes, there is plenty of insulin, but it is *ineffective* because it is *not allowed to act* due to *'resistance'* to its action. Unutilized insulin and sugar therefore keep accumulating in the blood. This excessive insulin is actually harmful and leads to a condition called 'metabolic syndrome' with disturbance in carbohydrate, protein and fat metabolism that leads to central obesity, Diabetes, high blood pressure, and increase in triglycerides (bad fats). You will understand better as you keep reading —

The story begins with resistance to action of insulin in muscles which is inherited or genetic. That means, muscles are unable to utilize sugar for their energy needs. Although insulin is ineffective, the *body thinks it is insufficient* — so more and more is secreted, and it keeps accumulating in the blood. High insulin levels chemically cause fat deposition in abdomen mainly in the omentum (see below) Omentum is a fold that hangs from the lower part of the stomach in the abdomen. —

Picture 1 and 2: — thin lace like omentum.

Picture 3: — solidified omentum with a lot of fat deposition.

Picture-4: — huge deposition of fat in omentum leading to ballooning of abdomen into 'apple shape'.

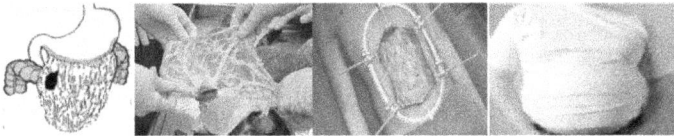

Omentum as you can see, is normally a net like, thin layer, containing some fat, but in some people excessive deposition leads to its getting solidified, filling up the abdomen giving it a bulging apple shape.

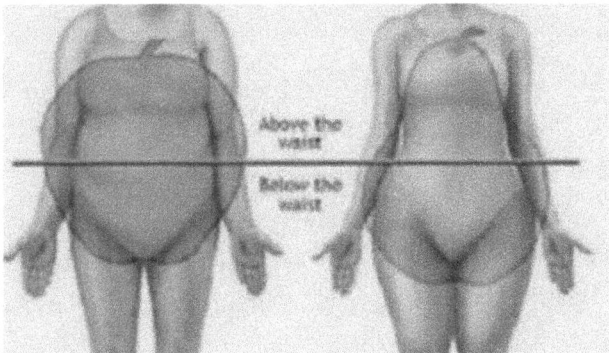

You can see that fat is deposited more above the waist. Conversely, in some people who are not prone to

Diabetes, fat is deposited below the waist giving the abdomen a 'pear shape' — so although apples are good for you, an apple shaped abdomen is not!

Excessive fat is also carried to liver where it gets deposited and interferes with action of insulin — which is to convert excess sugar from the blood into glycogen and store it for emergencies.. Again the body thinks insulin levels are *insufficient*, and the Pancreas is ordered to secrete more of it. So there is further increase in secretion of insulin to compensate the apparent deficiency.

Also fat in the form of triglycerols is released from the liver and carried to other organs, and especially to Pancreas. If you remember, Pancreas is the organ that secretes insulin from its Beta cells. *Fat deposit in the Pancreas interferes with release of insulin and also to a condition called 'apoptosis' or self-destruction and death of Beta cells. In fact removing as little as 1 gram of fat from the Pancreas can reverse Diabetes!* Let me give you the example of a thrifty housewife to explain the whole process.

- As soon as she receives some money in the beginning of the month, she keeps it for routine housekeeping expenses and school fees.

- If she receives some more money than is required for routine expenses, she keeps it in the cupboard for emergency expenditure during the month.

- If there is further surplus, she puts it into a bank FD.

- And if there is really a lot of money, she invests in shares/property.

- Now let us interpolate money with glucose. If the body receives some glucose, it utilizes it for energy (immediate expenses). When it receives more glucose than it can use, it stores it as glycogen in the liver (cupboard), to be converted into glucose whenever required. And if the glycogen stores are full, then excess sugar is converted into fat and stored in fat depots (banks). And lastly if even more sugar is available, it gets stored in Pancreas and liver as fat.(property/ shares).

- Now it is this extra fat deposition in the organs that leads to interference in action of insulin and Type II Diabetes.

At the time of diagnosis of Diabetes, most patients have already lost 50% of their Beta cells. Further destruction can be kept in check or at least slowed down by proper management of Diabetes. This should be your aim– *at any cost, keep your blood sugar under control, preserve your Beta cells, and prevent complications!* I think you are getting the hang of it by now – if not, go back and read again since it is important you understand *how* Diabetes occurs to be better able to manage it. In the next chapter you will learn about the common types and causes of Diabetes and whether it can be predicted and prevented.

Chapter 2

CAUSES, COMMON TYPES OF DIABETES, PRESENTATION, PREDICTING AND RISK FACTORS, HBA1C

There are many 'types' of Diabetes, but I am not going to bore you with all of them—the common ones are—

- **Type-1 Diabetes**—with absolute deficiency of insulin—normally seen in children and the young—there is a strong genetic base, and it is immune modulated.

- **Type 2 Diabetes**—with relative deficiency of insulin—mainly due to resistance to its action, normally seen after forty years of age—also a strong genetic base.

- **MODY**-There is a third type called MODY or maturity onset diabetes of young. This is also on the increase in children, since they are becoming sedentary, watching too much TV, with very little physical activity leading to adult type insulin resistance.

- **"Fibrocystic disease of the pancreas"** this is a disease where the pancreas gets destroyed in patients who are mal-nourished, and many thin diabetics after forty, have this acquired cause of diabetes. And another important type of diabetes is —

- **LADA** (Latent autoimmune diabetes in adults) — also called Type-1.5. LADA occurs in thin people after the age of forty and without other 'metabolic' features. LADA is important because these patients rapidly progress to insulin need after a few years of control with oral drugs. They therefore begin like Type -2 diabetes but rapidly progress to Type-I.

- **Other diseases of pancreas**

- **Drugs and chemicals** like Diuretics, some blood pressure lowering drugs, Hormones like birth control pills, steroids and thyroid hormones, anti psychotic medicines anti epileptic drugs, anti cancer drugs anti protozoal drugs (for intestinal infections). Other drugs are aspirin, statins (to lower bad fats) and theophylline (for Asthma).

- **Endocrinal diseases-**Hyperfunction of Adrenal, Thyroid and Pituitary glands can cause Diabetes

- **Gestational Diabetes —** diabetes during pregnancy.

If you have recently developed Diabetes, you should discuss with your doctor if any medication you are taking could have caused it, since withdrawing the drug may reverse your Diabetes. Your doctor will also rule out the diseases listed above that can cause Diabetes.

RISK FACTORS FOR DIABETES

Besides genetic factors, environmental factors are of utmost importance in causing diabetes mellitus. These include —

- Inappropriate dietary habits
- high bad fats in blood
- Obesity
- Lack of exercise
- High blood pressure
- Cigarette smoking
- Stress
- Immune reaction
- Viral infections
- All states that increase insulin requirements
- All states that decrease insulin formation in the Pancreas.

PRESENTATION OF DIABETES

There are a few common complaints by which diabetes presents itself like —

- Excessive urination
- Excessive thirst

- Excessive hunger
- Non-healing wounds
- Non-responding infections
- Complications of Diabetes, recent loss of weight can also be the presenting feature of Diabetes

PREDICTING DIABETES — can one predict Diabetes? There are a few indicators that can predict whether one will get diabetes —

- Positive genetic markers
- Obesity
- High omental fat
- Fatty infiltration liver on sonography
- Increase in pancreatic fat on sonography
- PCOD (Polycystic ovarian Disease) — in women
- Low C-peptide levels — the chemical that converts to insulin
- Low Serum insulin and pro-insulin levels
- Diseases of pancreas
- Endocrinal diseases
- Drug or chemical use that can cause Diabetes (see previous chapter)

TESTS FOR INSULIN RESISTANCE-there are special tests that can tell us if a person is suffering from insulin resistance, and is likely to get Type-11 diabetes in future.

- **HOMA** homeostatic model assessment
- **INSULIN LEVELS** in blood
- **INSULIN TOLERANCE TEST (ITT).**

This test involves an IV-infusion of insulin, with subsequent measurements of glucose and insulin levels.

- **QUICKI** Quantitative insulin sensitivity check index

PRE DIABETES

This is a condition in which Blood sugar is higher than normal but lower than in a Diabetic. These patients do not have symptoms of Diabetes but carry a high risk of becoming Diabetic. They also carry a 50% higher risk of heart disease and stroke.

Pre Diabetes can be diagnosed by these three tests —

- **Fasting blood glucose** — performed after an 8 hour fast —

Normal: Normal blood sugar levels measure less than 100 mg/dl (milligrams per deciliter) after the fasting glucose test.

Prediabetes : Blood glucose levels of 100-125 mg/dl after an overnight or eight-hour fast may indicate prediabetes. People with these results are considered to have impaired fasting glucose (IFG).

Diabetes: Diabetes is diagnosed when the blood glucose is 126 mg/dl or above after 8 hours of fasting.

- **Oral GTT**

After doing fasting blood glucose, 75 grams of glucose dissolved in water is given to the patient and blood glucose tested after 2 hours.

Normal: Normal blood sugar levels measure less than 140 mg/dl after 2 hours of consuming 75 grams of glucose.

Prediabetes: Blood glucose levels of 140-199 mg/dl after the OGTT is diagnosed as Prediabetes. People with these results are considered to have impaired glucose tolerance (IGT).

Diabetes: Diabetes is diagnosed with blood glucose of 200 mg/dl or above.

- **Random blood glucose** –140-200mgs is normal
- **HbA1c** – 4–5.7 % – normal
  5.7-6.4%–pre Diabetes
  >6.4% – Diabetes

Let me tell you a little more about this test–

GLYCOSELATED HAEMOGLOBIN – HBA1C

Glucose in the blood combines with haemoglobin –this is called glycoselated haemoglobin. Once glycoselated, this form of haemoglobin remains in the blood for about three months. This test is very important because it gives us an indication of *average blood glucose for the past three months* and a consistently high value is a warning of complications. *Results can be unreliable in many circumstances, such as after blood loss, after surgery, blood transfusions, anemia, high red cell turnover, in the presence* of chronic kidney or liver disease, after administration of high-dose vitamin C, or erythropoietin treatment that is given for anaemia in kidney failure.

The relationship between A1C and eAG (see below) is described by the formula 28.7 X A1C – 46.7 = eAG.

With this table you can get a rough idea of your HbA1C reading *from your three month home glucometer record.* Calculate average blood glucose after totaling all the readings and dividing by number of readings from last column—you can then match your HbA1c from first column.

HbA$_{1c}$		eAG (estimated average glucose)	
(%)	(mmol/mol)	(mmol/L)	(mg/dL)
5	31	5.4 (4.2–6.7)	97 (76–120)
6	42	7.0 (5.5–8.5)	126 (100–152)
7	53	8.6 (6.8–10.3)	154 (123–185)
8	64	10.2 (8.1–12.1)	183 (147–217)
9	75	11.8 (9.4–13.9)	212 (170–249)
10	86	13.4 (10.7–15.7)	240 (193–282)
11	97	14.9 (12.0–17.5)	269 (217–314)
12	108	16.5 (13.3–19.3)	298 (240–347)
13	119	18.1 (15–21)	326 (260–380)
14	130	19.7 (16–23)	355 (290–410)
15	140	21.3 (17–25)	384 (310–440)

HbA$_{1c}$		eAG (estimated average glucose)	
(%)	(mmol/ mol)	(mmol/L)	(mg/dL)
16	151	22.9 (19–26)	413 (330–480)
17	162	24.5 (20–28)	441 (460–510)
18	173	26.1 (21–30)	470 (380–540)
19	184	27.7 (23–32)	499 (410–570)

That was the end of Part I, next we go on to understand how to manage Diabetes, and the first chapter is naturally about do's and don'ts of diet.

PART II

MANAGEMENT OF DIABETES

CHAPTER 3

DIET IN DIABETES

BASICS

- To be built around a person's normal eating habits

- Small frequent meals

- Plenty of water and fluids (unsweetened, unsalted)

- Avoid red meat (high fat, no fibre)

- Avoid fats and fried foods

- Avoid fad diets — high protein, vegan

- Only 5tsf. Unsaturated oil a day (one tea-spoonful is 5 ml)

- Reduce sugar and salt

- Reduce maida, white bread, potatoes, polished rice

- 25 gms of fibre a day

- Avoid sweet fruits

- Include spices that burn fats – methi(fenugreek),haldi(turmeric), ginger, kali miri (black-pepper) –

Diet should be built around a person's normal eating habits

There is no single umbrella plan that works for all. Each patient's financial, cultural and employment status, and working conditions should be considered before designing a program tailored to his needs. Diet has to be individualized for each patient where a person's food preferences, cultural background, work schedule, and treatment goals have to be considered. General principles of Diet are given below from which a diet should be created.

You should eat small, frequent four- hourly meals to avoid a load on the pancreas. A thin diabetic can take more calories but an obese diabetic has to restrict calories according to his body weight.

What to avoid

- Simple sugars like sugar (unrefined sugar), honey, all sweets, maida (refined flour) products (maida biscuits, white bread) potatoes and white rice.
- Sweet fruits –like bananas, mangoes, custard apple, chickoos and grapes.
- Above foods have a 'high glycaemic index', that is they cause sugar to rise rapidly in blood.
- Saturated fats– like ghee, butter, cheese and dalda.
- Red meat, egg-yolk

What to eat

Plenty of vegetables, a bowl of mixed salads, a small cup of mixed sprouts, three cups of skimmed milk, 3 cups skimmed milk curds, all pulses(lentils) and legumes, fish, whole grain chapattis, red/unpolished rice, any one bitter, less sweet fruits like citrus fruits, berries, pomegranate, papaya, grape-fruit, and *Stevia* and *sucralose* containing artificial sweeteners (minimal amounts).

Chapattis and bread should be made from whole meal and preferably multigrain cereals.

Bitters should be incorporated in the diet – like methi (fenugreek), karela (bitter gourd), neem etc. which seem to help in controlling blood sugar and also bring down cholesterol.

Proteins, carbohydrates, fats

5% calories should come from saturated fats

15% calories from unsaturated fats—Rice bran oil, soya, nuts, olives, olive oil, canola

oil, mustard and Til (sesame oils)

25-30% calories from protein—fish, egg white, grains, pulses and legumes

Rest of the calories from–complex carbohydrates (whole wheat and bajra, besan, brown rice, low fat milk, low fat curds.

Brown bread, sprouts, whole pulses, legumes, salads, fruits, whole wheat cereal, cornflakes, oats, boiled egg white, paneer, roasted chana, wheat and bajra-murmura, besan-cheela(made of gram flour), isabgol,– are good foods for diabetics.

Milk should preferably be skimmed.

Vegetables – all except potatoes – you can eat potatoes in moderation – cook with skin, and add a little with other vegetables.

Summary of Diet

Free foods – (Take any amount) –Plain Tea, coffee, Lemon juice (Nimboo Pani,) clear soup, khatti lassi,(buttermilk) kheera (kakdi, cucumber) Tomato, Mooli, (radish) Karela (bitter gourd) & Leafy vegetables.

Foods allowed

Cereals	-	un-sieved wheat flour, daliya, (broken wheat) and bajra, jowar ragi (millets), unpolished rice, boiled rice, rice with starch drained out.
Pulses	-	all pulses & sprouts allowed
Vegetables	-	all except, potato, arvi (colocasia),beet- root (take less)
Fruits	-	apples, cherries, guava, lemon, sweet lime, water- melon, melon, orange, papaya, pear, pineapple, pomegranate, strawberry, jamun (blue berries), and all other berries can be taken in small helpings three to five times a day. Preferably combine with sprouts and salads to reduce glycaemic index.

Oil	-	mustard, til, olive, rice bran, soya
Chicken	-	thrice a week (without skin)
Fish	-	180 grams twice a week

Foods to be restricted — (not totally avoided).

Whole milk, whole milk curds, butter, ghee,(clarified butter) cheese, khoa,(concentrated milk) coconuts, pickles, fried foods, alcohol.

Foods to be avoided

Mainly avoid–Sugar, sweets, cakes, pastries, honey, brown sugar, sweetened juices, dates, processed foods (contain corn syrup).

White rice, rice-flakes, refined flours, white bread, sago, Arrowroot, Potato, and other underground vegetables, besides mangoes, bananas, chickoos, grapes, sitaphal (custard apple) .

Fibre : It is a very important ' waste ' product of food and an essential component of our daily food intake. It can be water soluble or insoluble –

Soluble Fibre: Soluble fibre, holds water to form a gel - like fenugreek, barley, plums, raisins, beans, isapgol, (natural husk) carrots and guar gum etc.

Uses: Consuming enough soluble fibre, gives a feeling of fullness (thereby reducing food intake), softens our stools, and delays absorption of sugar into the blood.

Insoluble fibre: It is found in skins, peels, seeds and husks of fruits and vegetables as also in whole grains.

Uses: It provides bulk to food, softens stools, and traps and throws out fats. Fibre, thus has zero calories, helps in constipation, diarrhoea, weight reduction, diabetes, hyperlipidaemia (increase in bad fats), piles, and even prevents bowel cancer.

So make sure you consume daily five hundred grams of fruits and vegetables, and always eat whole grain cereals so that your body gets enough of this useful substance unfortunately called a 'waste '.

Hardly a waste product don't you agree!

Next we talk about a fibre-rich and nutri-rich entity called — sprouts.

Just see what happens when we sprout a seed, whole pulse or legume —

SPROUTS THE NUTRITIONAL WONDER

Caloric content	reduced 15%
Carbohydrate content	reduced 15-30%
Protein content	increased 30%
B complex vitamins	increased 200- 500%
Calcium	increased 34 %
Iron	increased 40%
Potassium	increased 80%
Phosphorous	increased 56%
Vitamin A	increased 285%
Vitamin C	infinite increase
Salt?	slightly increased

All seeds sesame, groundnuts, melon seeds, flax seeds, sunflower seeds), lentils (whole pulses), and legumes (whole) can be sprouted.

Examples of legumes are peas, dried beans, chick-peas, small black eyed peas etc. But make sure you sprout them at home and use clean water, so that you do not pick up an infection!

Most of the benefits are obtained on consuming raw sprouts.

Chew thoroughly and eat to get almost all your vitamins, minerals, proteins and fibre requirements! You will have seen a question mark after 'salt'—yes, salt content is also increased so reduce your salt intake if you are regularly consuming sprouts.

Some common artificial sweeteners or sugar substitutes

With the availability of artificial sweeteners, diabetics can lead a sweeter life and these can be used imaginatively to make sweets or added to beverages. But make sure you use them within limits.

- *Saccharin*

Saccharin is 300-500 times sweeter than sugar but leaves a bitter after taste and some experiments on rats have shown that it can lead to cancer. Although its safety has been proved in human beings, it is not very popular these days.

- *Aspartame*

Aspartame is about 200 times as sweet as sugar. When cooked or stored at high temperatures, aspartame breaks down into its constituent amino acids and loses its sweetness. Therefore it cannot be added during cooking or to foods and beverages that are heated. It is considered safe for human consumption.

- *Stevia*

Stevia is a herbal product that has been used for centuries in South America, and now all over the world. It is safe for human consumption.

- *Lactulose*

Lactulose is a sweetener that is a mild laxative and is also used to remove toxic ammonia from the blood in those with liver failure. Most of it is not absorbed, but broken down to acids that create an osmotic effect, drawing water into the intestines — thus increasing stool bulk. But some amount is broken down into fructose and galactose; which may be absorbed and increase blood sugar.

- *Sucralose*

Sucralose is a chlorinated sugar that is 600 times as sweet as sugar. It is produced from sucrose (sugar) and most of it passes out unabsorbed from the body. That is why it does not add to calorie intake. It is safe for human consumption. But recent studies are showing it can alter the natural bacterial flora content in the intestines, which can actually interfere with action of insulin — so limit your intake to the minimum.

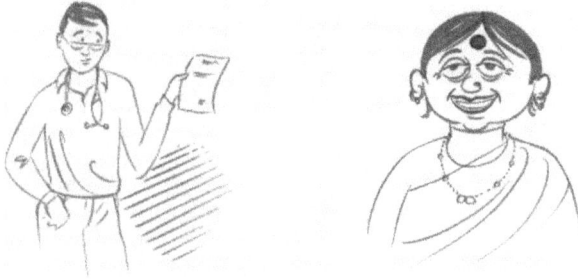

Glycaemic index

Glycaemic index is a term used to measure glycaemic response—that is how quickly a food item gets converted into sugar and enters the blood stream in comparison to an equivalent amount of sugar. Foods are therefore classified into low and high glycaemic substances.

GI of glucose is taken to be 100 (maximum). The closer the GI of different foods to glucose (high GI), the more unsafe it is for a diabetic. Conversely low GI foods are safe for consumption by a diabetic.

A high GI value is 70 or more
A medium GI value is 56-69
A low GI value is less than 55

If you see different glycaemic index tables, you will find varying values for the same foods. This is because of different methods of testing, portion sizes used and also because the carbohydrate, protein and fat content of the same food may vary from place to place. For example the amylase content of white rice can vary so much that the glycaemic index of white rice can be depicted anywhere from 90-100. It is therefore important to understand the general guidelines for glycaemic index. The following tables will give you an idea of GI of various foods, but before that a special mention of rice —

White rice (polished) has a GI of 90 — 100.

Basmati rice — around 65 -70

Par boiled rice — around 67

Brown unpolished rice — 48

So brown rice is best since it has the highest amount of fiber, selenium that prevents aging, omega-3 fatty acids that are good for heart and brain, vitamin E that keeps us young, and lastly vitamin B-1 that is good for nerves.

Parboiled rice is rice that is boiled to 70 degrees and quickly cooled. This pushes all the useful nutrients into the rice from the bran which is then removed. So par boiled rice is nutrient rich but lacks fiber.

Next is Basmati rice that lacks the nutrients but has a lower GI than white rice and has the best flavour. Brown basmati is better than polished basmati but not as good as ordinary brown rice.

Last is polished white rice especially the sticky type — with highest GI, no nutrients, and no fiber.

Draining out starch reduces GI but you lose out on all nutrients. So pressure cook your rice to retain nutrients.

There are other types of rice like red and black — but since they are rare, I am not discussing here.

Bananas, mangoes, grapes and Diabetes

Slightly unripe and smaller bananas have lower GI (around 32) – can be eaten. Riper and larger ones have higher GI (54-70).

Eat small helpings of mangoes — choose half ripe –GI 50 — (fully ripe GI is around 70), grapes (GI 48-50).

Some high GI foods — (bad) Sugar, sweets, cakes, pastries, honey, brown sugar, sweetened juices, dates, white rice, rice-flakes, refined flours, white bread, sago, Arrowroot, Potato, sweet- potato, and other underground vegetables, besides mangoes, chickoos, sitaphal (custard apple) .

Some low GI foods(good)

Sprouts, whole pulses, legumes, salads, fruits, boiled egg white, paneer,(cottage cheese) roasted chana(chick peas), wheat and bajra (millet) murmura, besan(chick peas flour) cheela, isabgol, rajma,(kidney beans) peanuts, chana,(chick peas) brown rice, low fat milk, low fat curds, apples.

If you eat a high GI food, combine it with a large portion of low GI food to balance out. For example if you want to eat poha(flattened rice) — add a lot of methi leaves or peas to lower the GI.

Table 1 - Low GI Foods

Food	GI
Peanuts	14
Low-fat yoghurt	14
Cherries	22
Grapefruit	25
Pearl barley	25
Red lentils(rajma)	26
Whole milk	27
beans	31
Skimmed milk	32
Wholemeal spaghetti, noodles	37
Apples	38
Pears	38
Tomato soup	38
Apple juice, unsweetened	40
White spaghetti	41
Kabuli chana(chick peas)	42
Peaches	42
Porridge made with water	42
Lentil soup(dal)	44
Oranges	44
Macaroni	45
Green grapes	46
Orange juice	46
Peas	48
Baked beans in tomato sauce	48
Unpolished or brown rice	48
Carrots, boiled	49
Milk chocolate	49
wholemeal bread	53

Table 2 Medium Glycaemic Index foods (55 to 69)

Banana	55
Raw oat bran	55
Sweet corn	55
Muesli	56
Boiled potatoes	56
Basmati Rice, boiled rice	58
Honey	58
Cheese and tomato pizza	60
Ice cream	61
New potatoes	62
Coca cola	63
Raisins	64
Pineapple, fresh	66
Melon	67
Shredded wheat	67
Whole meal bread	69

Table 3 High Glycaemic Index foods (70 or more)

Avoid totally or combine with low GI foods

Mashed potato	70
White bread	70
Watermelon	72
French fries	75
Rice cakes	82
Cornflakes	84
Jacket potato	85
Puffed wheat	89
White rice, steamed	98

Glycaemic load — how to reduce glycaemic index of common Indian foods

--Do not grind food fine, do not overcook;

--- Add low glycaemic foods, and vegetables to reduce glycaemic load of high GI foods

Upma, poha, rice — add plenty of vegetables

Idli, dosa, dhokla — add more pulses, methi seeds, vegetables, flax seed, use brown or boiled rice and do not grind very fine

Parathas and chappattis — add vegetables, soya, isabgol, bajra, barley

Muthia — add vegetables, methi, flax seed

Dals — add vegetables

Medicinal plants that help in diabetes

Fenugreek or Methi

The seed of Fenugreek contains the most potent medicinal effects of the plant. It is primarily used for preventing hardening of arteries, diabetes, and triglycerides (bad fats) and also helps in constipation. It can be taken 5-30 grams with each meal or 15-90 grams all at once with one meal. It can be soaked overnight and consumed or as powders, or as sprouts. Use of more than 100 grams of fenugreek seeds daily can cause intestinal upset and nausea. Otherwise, fenugreek is safe.

Neem

Following are said to be some of the exciting uses for neem besides Diabetes — Psoriasis, AIDS, Cancer, Heart disease, periodontal disease, Ulcers.

Basil (Tulsi)

Holy Basil called Tulsi in Indian language originated in India, and is planted in mostly all Hindu homes, as it is treated as a holy plant. Besides its religious reasons, It improves overall health in Diabetes. Consuming Tulsi leaf everyday also is said to prevent cough, cold, fever, flu, disorders of stomach, throat, nose, teeth and eyes.

Others — turmeric (haldi), kala jeera (black cumin), and jamun (blueberry)seed powder are also said to lower blood glucose.

Sweets and diabetes —

When your craving for sweets is high----indulge yourself with a small helping of sugar free sweets!

You are only human, and sometimes the craving for sweets can hit you — during these times, you can take a small helping of sweets made from sucralose or stevia. Examples are — sugar free ice-cream, kheer and halwas with dried figs (anjir), dried dates (khajur), raisins (kismis). Try to use less of artificial sweeteners and more of sweet dry fruits. But do remember to take small helpings and once in a while only.

Make kheer ,halwas and puddings as usual and add these natural sweet dry fruits to taste. You can also make barfis, and laddoos. Here are some interesting recipes —

Pooran poli

Make dough with milk,whole wheat, kesar(saffron) and ilaichi (cardamom) powder. Make chana dal pooran as usual and mix with mashed dates and kismis(raisins). Add grated fresh coconut. Roll out polis, stuff pooran, reroll and sauté on tawa with a little oil.

Choorma laddoo

Take two cups whole wheat flour, add 4 tsf hot ghee(clarified butter), 6 tsf milk, Mix everything and make small flat rounds. Then microwave for 3-5 mts. Remove, crumble fine, and add 6 dates de-seeded, ¼ cup kismis(raisins),some ilaichi powder, and 1 tsf hot ghee. Mix well and make laddoos.

Sugar free kulfi

Take equal quantities of milk powder and coconut milk powder. Add cocoa powder one tablespoonful (or any other flavor) if you want. Add enough milk to liquefy. Add a little sugar free natura/Diet sugar to taste. Stir till thick. Pour into moulds and freeze.

Carrot/Tomato barfi

Take 4 carrots grated or tomatoes diced small, plus 2 tablespoons of rava or oats and cook in 2tsf ghee. Add 2 tablespoons of milk powder, four dried anjir (figs), 8 dates and some ilaichi (cardamom) powder.

Cook till it becomes solid, remove in a greased plate and cut into barfis.

Any barfi

Take a cup of khoya (concentrated milk)and stir on low flame till it begins to melt. Add ingredient of any barfi — coconut, pista, kaju,(cashew) badaam(almonds) etc, and sugar free natura to taste.(or sweeten with raisins/dates or figs) Stir till solid, pour into container, cool and cut into shapes.

Chocolate barfi-

8-10 sugar free oats or ragi biscuits crumbled, add half cup milk, 100 grams dried coconut powder, half cup ghee, 2 tablespoons sugar free, and 2 tablespoons cocoa powder. Stir till solid, remove from fire, pour into greased plate, cool in fridge and then cut into pieces.

Sugar free biscuits

Take multigrain atta (flour) 3 cups, 8-10 edible gond (ding, edible gum — made to swell up in microwave or on gas — then crumbled), half cup melted ghee,(clarified butter) 6 tsf dried date powder, 1 tsf dried ginger powder, half spoon baking powder, half spoon soda, quarter spoon salt, 4 tsf sugar free powder (optional). Mix well, make into flat biscuit shapes and microwave.

As important as diet is exercise in controlling Diabetes, which we will discuss in the next chapter.

CHAPTER 4

EXERCISE

Exercise is important to keep weight under control and also to help in more efficient utilization of sugar.

Moderate exercise – aerobic and anaerobic should be actively encouraged in all diabetics. *Five kilometers of walk or five thousand steps a day are ideal. You can use a smart phone or pedometer or count your steps once to know you have walked 5 km. You can also do it in 10 minute spurts throughout day.* Approximately 1400-1500 steps make a kilometer — depending on your height and stride.

Maintain adequate hydration before, during and after sustained exercise.

Patients with moderate and severe type 2 diabetes should be advised not to drink alcohol at night if they plan to exercise the following morning.

- You should select appropriate fitting shoes for exercise.

- Socks also should fit well and be made from material that absorbs moisture to keep the feet dry.

- Symptoms of dizziness, weakness, or shortness of breath should be an alert for the possibility of heart disease. If you have any of these complaints, you should undertake a stress test and have monitored exercise sessions.

> • Symptoms of dizziness, weakness, or shortness of breath should be an alert for the possibility of cardiac disease.

- Those of you who have retinopathy (involvement of screen behind eye) should be wary of high intensity activities that can cause bleeding in eye or retinal detachment.

- Non-weight-bearing activities or specially modified footwear should be considered for those of you with peripheral nerve involvement, so as to reduce trauma to the lower legs and feet.

- If your fasting sugar is less than 100mg% take carbohydrates (a small chappati, a slice of brown bread) before exercising

- Those of you with kidney involvement should avoid strenuous activities

- Do not exercise if — systolic blood pressure is above 200mm Hg/100mm or FBG more than 250mg%

How exercise helps

- Decreases risk of heart disease

- Reduces body fat stores

- Improves glucose utilization

- Enhances fitness

- Reduces stress

Ha Ha!

You can suffer from good health by exercising daily or enjoy Diabetes and blood pressure lifelong!

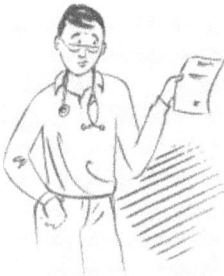

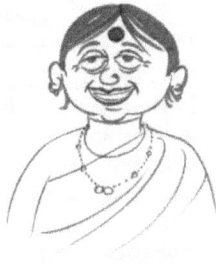

ACSM (American college of sports medicine) recommendations

If you are performing high intensity exercise, 3 days of exercise per week will yield the desired results.

If you are performing low intensity exercise you may require daily exercise

If you are performing high intensity exercise 5 to 6 days per week you should avoid overtraining and overuse injuries.

Activities such as walking, hiking, jogging, running, cycling, swimming, rowing, dancing, skating etc can all be used to improve cardio respiratory fitness.

Sports such as racquetball, handball, football and basketball are also effective provided they are played at high intensity for an adequate duration.

Exercise in patients with loss of protective sensation in the feet-

Avoid–

- Treadmill
- Prolonged walking
- Jogging
- Step exercises

Can do–

- Swimming
- Bicycling
- Rowing
- Chair exercises
- Upper body exercises
- Other non-weight-bearing exercise

Resistance exercise

Resistance exercises with weights, bands or machines) are useful for building adequate muscular strength and endurance.

1. Choose a mode of exercise (free weights, bands, machines) that is comfortable through a pain-free range of motion.

2. Perform 8 to 10 exercises that train the major muscles of the hips, thigh, legs, back, chest, shoulders, arms and abdomen. Perform 1 set of each exercise till voluntary fatigue.

3. Exercise each muscle group on 2 to 3 non-consecutive days of the week.

4. Adhere as closely as possible to the specific techniques for performing a given exercise.

5. Give enough recovery time between 2 exercises.

6. Perform the lifting (concentric) and lowering (eccentric) phases of the exercise in a controlled manner.

7. Always keep small weights or a dumb-bell near you while watching TV and keep doing resistance exercises for upper body—hands, elbow, shoulder, etc.

8. Breathe normally during lifting because breath holding can increase blood pressure.

Remember when you tire out mentally and physically —

TODAY IT HURTS — TOMORROW IT WORKS!

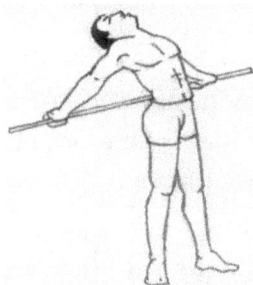

YOUR BODY CAN DO ANYTHING — JUST CONVINCE YOUR MIND!

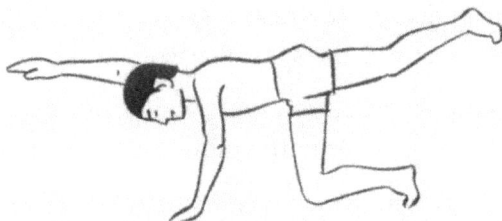

The next important arm of Diabetes management is to reach and maintain ideal body weight. You will learn how to do this in the next chapter.

CHAPTER 5

CONTROL OF BODY WEIGHT

You should aim for ideal body weight (see chart below). In fact it is a good idea to keep it 10% below normal.

The primary approach for achieving weight loss is lifestyle change, which includes a reduction in energy intake and an increase in physical activity. Weight loss diets should supply at least 1000-1200 kcal/day for women and 1200-1600 kcal/day for men.

All diabetics should aim for ideal body weight or 10% below that

STANDARD HEIGHT & WEIGHT FOR INDIAN MEN & WOMEN

HEIGHT	WEIGHT (MEN) Kg	WEIGHT (WOMEN) Kg
1.52M(5'-0")	-	50-54
1.54M(5'-1")	-	51-55
1.57M(5'-2")	56-60	53-56

1.59M(5'-3")	57-61	54-58
1.62M(5'-4")	59-63	56-60
1.65M(5'-5")	61-65	58-61
1.67M(5'-6")	62-67	59-64
1.70M(5'-7")	64-68	61-65
1.72M(5'-8")	66-71	62-67
1.75M(5'-9")	68-73	64-69
1.77M(5'-10")	69-74	66-70
1.80M(5'-11")	71-76	67-72
1.82M(6'-0")	73-78	69-74
1.85M(6'-1")	75-81	-
1.87M(6'-2")	77-84	-
Source: Life Insurance Corporation of India		

BODY MASS INDEX

B M I is a good index of obesity. It is calculated by dividing body weight in kg by height in meters squared. All Diabetics should aim for normal BMI.

B M I
Less than 25	- normal
25 - 30	- is over weight
More than 30	- is obese

	Good	**Normal**	**Increased**
Males	below 25	25-27	above27
Females	below 23	23-25	above25

Males should aim for a BMI below 27, and females, below 25

BODY MASS INDEX

		Height (cm)									
		145	150	155	160	165	170	175	180	185	190
Weight (Kg)	50	24	22	21	20	18	17	16	15	15	14
	52	25	23	22	20	19	18	17	16	15	14
	54	26	24	22	21	20	19	18	17	16	15
	56	27	25	23	22	21	19	18	17	16	16
	58	28	26	24	23	21	20	19	18	17	16
	60	29	27	25	23	22	21	20	19	18	17
	62	29	28	26	24	23	21	20	19	18	17
	64	30	28	27	25	24	22	21	20	19	18
	66	31	29	27	26	24	23	22	20	19	18
	68	32	30	28	27	25	24	22	21	20	19
	70	33	31	29	27	26	24	23	22	20	19
	72	34	32	30	28	26	25	24	22	21	20
	74	35	33	31	29	27	26	24	23	22	20
	76	36	34	32	30	28	26	25	23	22	21
	78	37	35	32	30	29	27	25	24	23	22
	80	38	36	33	31	29	28	26	25	23	22
	82	39	36	34	32	30	28	27	25	24	23
	84	40	37	35	33	31	29	27	26	25	23
	86	41	38	36	34	32	30	28	27	25	24
	88	42	39	37	34	32	30	29	27	26	24
	90	43	40	37	35	33	31	29	28	26	25

Another important measurement is waist hip ratio that needs to be kept normal. Waist circumference at umbilicus in cms divided by hip circumference in cms = W H R

WAIST HIP RATIO

W H R

More than 0.95   - is abdominal obesity in males

More than 0.85   - is abdominal obesity in females

HIP MEASUREMENT cms

WAIST MEASURMENT (cms.)

140	135	130	125	120	115	110	105	100	95	90	85	80	75	70	65	60	55	50	HIP
2.80	2.70	2.60	2.50	2.40	2.30	2.20	2.10	2.00	1.90	1.80	1.70	1.60	1.50	1.40	1.30	1.20	1.10	1.00	50
2.55	2.45	2.36	2.27	2.18	2.09	2.00	1.91	1.82	1.73	1.64	1.55	1.45	1.36	1.27	1.18	1.09	1.00	0.91	55
2.33	2.25	2.17	2.08	2.00	1.92	1.83	1.75	1.67	1.58	1.50	1.42	1.33	1.25	1.17	1.08	1.00	0.92	0.83	60
2.15	2.08	2.00	1.92	1.85	1.77	1.69	1.62	1.54	1.46	1.38	1.31	1.23	1.15	1.08	1.00	0.92	0.85	0.77	65
2.00	1.93	1.86	1.79	1.71	1.67	1.57	1.50	1.43	1.36	1.29	1.21	1.14	1.07	1.00	0.93	0.86	0.79	0.71	70
1.87	1.80	1.73	1.67	1.60	1.53	1.47	1.40	1.33	1.27	1.20	1.13	1.07	1.00	0.93	0.87	0.80	0.73	0.67	75
1.75	1.69	1.63	1.56	1.50	1.44	1.38	1.31	1.25	1.19	1.13	1.06	1.00	0.94	0.88	0.81	0.75	0.69	0.63	80
1.65	1.59	1.53	1.47	1.41	1.35	1.29	1.24	1.18	1.12	1.06	1.00	0.94	0.88	0.82	0.76	0.71	0.65	0.59	85
1.56	1.50	1.44	1.39	1.33	1.28	1.22	1.17	1.11	1.06	1.00	0.94	0.89	0.83	0.87	0.72	0.67	0.61	0.56	90
1.47	1.42	1.37	1.32	1.26	1.21	1.16	1.11	1.05	1.00	0.95	0.89	0.84	0.79	0.74	0.68	0.63	0.58	0.53	95
1.40	1.35	1.30	1.25	1.20	1.15	1.10	1.05	1.00	0.95	0.90	0.85	0.80	0.75	0.70	0.65	0.60	0.55	0.50	100
1.33	1.29	1.24	1.19	1.14	1.10	1.05	1.00	0.95	0.90	0.86	0.81	0.76	0.71	0.67	0.62	0.57	0.52	0.48	105
1.27	1.23	1.18	1.14	1.09	1.05	1.00	0.95	0.91	0.86	0.82	0.77	0.73	0.68	0.64	0.59	0.55	0.50	0.45	110
1.22	1.17	1.13	1.09	1.04	1.00	0.96	0.91	0.87	0.83	0.78	0.74	70.0	0.65	0.61	0.57	0.52	0.48	0.43	115
1.17	1.13	1.08	1.04	1.00	0.96	0.92	0.88	0.83	0.79	0.75	0.71	0.67	0.63	0.58	0.54	0.50	0.46	0.42	120
1.12	1.08	1.04	1.00	0.96	0.92	0.88	0.84	0.80	0.76	0.72	0.68	0.64	0.60	0.56	0.52	0.48	0.44	0.40	125
1.08	1.04	1.00	0.96	0.92	0.88	0.85	0.81	0.77	0.73	0.69	0.65	0.62	0.58	0.54	0.50	0.46	0.42	0.38	130
1.04	1.00	0.96	0.93	0.89	0.85	0.81	0.78	0.74	0.70	0.67	0.63	0.59	0.56	0.52	0.48	0.44	0.41	0.37	135
1.00	0.96	0.93	0.89	0.88	0.82	0.79	0.75	0.71	0.68	0.64	0.61	0.57	0.54	0.50	0.46	0.43	0.39	0.36	140
0.97	0.93	0.90	0.86	0.83	0.79	0.76	0.72	0.69	0.68	0.62	0.59	0.55	0.52	0.48	0.45	0.41	0.38	0.34	145
0.93	0.90	0.87	0.83	0.80	0.77	0.73	0.70	0.67	0.63	0.60	0.57	0.53	0.50	0.47	0.43	0.40	0.37	0.33	150

WHR should be below 0.95 in males and below 0.85 in females and is in fact a more important risk factor than IBW or BMI.

Waist height ratio/ Waist circumference

But the single and most important measurement in a Diabetic is the waist circumference and a simple formula to use is that it should be less than half your height in centimeters. For example if your height is 170 cms your waist circumference should be less than 85 cms. All you need is an inch tape – measure the girth of the waist just above the hips at the umbilicus, without compressing the abdomen – that's it! Keep track of this and maintain the ratio of waist to height less than 0.5 cms – and your Diabetes will be under control.

WAIST CIRCUMFERENCE

CATEGORY	INTERNATIONAL MEN	INTERNATIONAL WOMEN	ASIAN/ INDIAN-MEN	ASIAN/ INDIAN-WOMEN
NORMAL	<100 cms	<90 cms	<90 cms	<80 cms
To avoid Diabetes			<78 cms	<72 cms

How much exercise?

You should gradually increase the duration and frequency to 30 to 45 min of moderate aerobic activity, 3 to 5 days/week (goal at least 150min/wk). Greater activity levels of at least 1 hr/day of moderate(walking)/uphill walking, or 30 min/day of vigorous (jogging) activity may be needed to achieve successful long-term weight loss. Drug therapy for obesity and surgery to induce weight loss maybe appropriate in selected patients.

There are four steps in losing weight —

- Diet
- Exercise
- Behavioral methods
- Artificial methods

Diet and exercise have already been discussed —

Behavioral methods for losing weight

- Disturbance in body image of self should be corrected

- *Availability* of high calorie food should be restricted

- Time of eating should be delayed
- Food should be eaten slowly (at least 20 mts) — to stimulate satiety center with least amount of food.
- Partying, feasting, watching too much T.V. should be reduced
- Group therapy to motivate each other
- Movement- keep moving to burn calories
- Ask yourself every time — do I really need to eat this?
- Stop buying processed foods from outside
- Avoid eating out as far as possible

Offer guests healthy juices and food when you invite them home

Artificial measures –

- **Appetite suppressants-**
    - *High fibre powders-*too much can interfere with absorption of essential nutrients–total fibre intake should not exceed 25 grams a day.
    - *High protein powders-* have been known to cause heart enlargement in USA.
    - **Drugs-** like sibutramine (lowers appetite) and orlistat (reduces fat absorption by body) — take under medical supervision.

- **Herbal preparations**–which "burn" fat–take them with caution under supervision of qualified doctor.

- **Liposuction**–to remove fat selectively from some areas–should be performed only by very experienced cosmetic surgeons & in limited quantities only, so as not to endanger life.

- **Surgery** to reduce size of stomach — by bypassing part of the stomach, tying a band to part of the stomach,(almost obsolete) or cutting off a sleeve from the stomach and stapling the remaining active portion. Some examples are given below as pictures —

Roux – en – Y Gastric Bypass **Banded Gastroplasty**

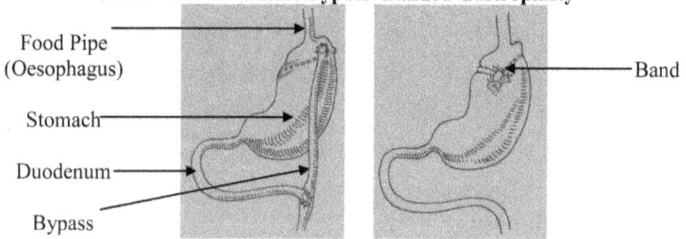

Food Pipe (Oesophagus)

Stomach

Duodenum

Bypass

Band

Sleeve gastrectomy

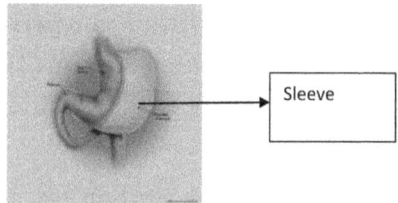

Sleeve

It is also important to keep your blood pressure and bad fats under control to avoid complications — we will learn how in the next chapter.

CHAPTER 6

Other measures in management

Control of blood pressure

Controlling blood pressure reduces chances of complications developing in a diabetic. This can be achieved by reducing intake of salt, keeping lipids under control (see below), exercise, maintaining ideal body weight, taking medication regularly and going for check-ups.

DIET IN HYPERTENSION-

Salt

Our body actually requires only 2000 milligrams of salt in a day from food, which can increase in summer, but most of us consume 30-50 times that amount. Try to avoid highly salted and preserved foods like pickles and salted snacks. On the other hand *calcium, magnesium and potassium* keep the blood pressure low. Normal salt contains 40% *sodium.* You can use low sodium salts available in the market, which contain only 18 % sodium. But this should be avoided if you have kidney failure since it contains high potassium levels which are harmful in this condition.

Potassium

Best source of potassium are fruits.

Calcium

Greens and dairy products supply enough calcium.

Magnesium

Magnesium is present in nuts, sprouts Soya beans and bananas.

Diet for hypertension should therefore be vegetarian (plus fish), high in fibre, a lot of fruits (they provide fibre and potassium), plenty of vegetables (fibre and calcium), avoidance of solid fats (ghee, butter, margarine, cheese), and less of refined foods like refined flour, sugar etc

The **DASH diet** (**D**ietary **A**pproaches to **S**top **H**ypertension)

This is a dietary pattern promoted by the U.S.-based National Heart, Lung, and Blood Institute to prevent and control hypertension. The DASH diet is rich in fruits, vegetables, whole grains, and low-fat dairy foods; includes fish, poultry, nuts and beans; and is limited in sugar-sweetened foods and beverages, red meat, and added fats. In addition to its effect on blood pressure, it is considered a well-balanced approach to eating for the general public. It is now recommended by the US Department of Agriculture (USDA) as an ideal eating plan for all Americans. The US Dietary Guidelines for Americans recommend eating a diet of 2300 mg of sodium a day or lower, with a recommendation of 1500 mg/day in adults who have elevated blood pressure; the 1500 mg/day is the low sodium level tested in the DASH-Sodium study.

At sodium intake level of 1,500 mg/day, plus the other recommendations of DASH diet, there was reduction in blood pressure which was in fact equal to that achieved by a single drug for lowering blood pressure.

> BP should be kept below 130/80 in a Diabetic

Control of lipids

Fats are made up of fatty acids which may be EFA (essential fatty acids) which cannot be synthesized by the body & have to be supplied from outside, & NEFA (non essential fatty acids) which are synthesized by the body. Fats can also be classified into SAFA, PUFA, or MUFA —

- SAFA (saturated fatty acids) — ghee (clarified butter), butter, mayonnaise, coconut oil and margarine, contain saturated fatty acids and should be avoided.

Hydrogenation of vegetable oils leads to their solidification thus increasing their shelf life but in the process, destroying nutrients, with addition of TFA (Trans fatty acids), which interfere with formation of EFA (essential or good fatty acids) in the body. Example.of hydrogenated oils are- Margarine.

- PUFA (poly unsaturated fatty acids) This may be PUFA –6 or PUFA –3

Pufa- 3 fatty acids are good for the heart (*also called omega –3 or essential fatty acids*) and are present in rice-bran, fish, soya and rape seed oils and to some extent in other unsaturated oils. They are also present in green leafy vegetables, sprouts, & algae. Omega –3 fatty acids are not only good for the heart, but also required for proper functioning of the brain.

- MUFA (Mono unsaturated fatty acids) are *good for the heart*& present in olive, canola, dark green leafy vegetables, & nuts like peanuts, almonds, cashew, etc.

We can achieve correct balance of these oils by taking a mixture of oils, like peanut, mustard, sunflower, Soya, sesame, rice-bran and safflower oil. Or we can alternate usage of these oils every month.

Bad lipids can also be lowered by taking at least 25 grams of fibre a day. Lipid lowering drugs may also be required in those with severe problems.

Among the unsaturated oils - rice bran oil, Soya, fish oil and rapeseed oil– are best for the you. We do not use fish and rapeseed oil as cooking media. Mustard, til (sesame), soya, rice-bran, and olive oil are good. Corn, groundnut (peanut), and sunflower are also O.K in moderation. Virgin olive oil should not be used for cooking—only for salad dressing, since harmful disease causing trans fatty acids are created if it is heated. Use a combination of these and try to use as many as you can. One or two can be used as cooking media, according to your preference, and the others can be consumed as powders added during cooking. e.g. – mustard, sesame and pea nut powders. A good method is to alternate type of oil used so that you get benefits of different oils.

Don't get carried away by advertisements showing particular oils being used to fry food, and proclaiming such fried food, are *good* for you! The main point is not only *which oil* but also *how much* of it, since excessive intake of *any oil* will make us put on weight and there can be nothing worse for the you than obesity. Stick to 5 teaspoonfuls of oil a day of your choice and use something like rice bran oil for occasionally frying.

Regularity

Remember to be regular in your eating habits, exercise, medicine intake and check-ups.

Regular Monitoring and regular check-ups are of tremendous significance to make sure diabetic control is maintained smoothly, preventing complications and for adjustments in dosage of medications.

Stress is something that can precipitate Diabetes if you are already prone to it and also make it difficult to keep under control. So you must learn to handle stress. Learn how in the next chapter.

CHAPTER 7

STRESS AND DIABETES

If there is one factor that really harms you as a Diabetic, it is stress. Let us understand stress and how it affects a Diabetic

Can we define stress? Put simply, we can call it a "force, pressure or strain exerted upon a person who resists these forces without attempting to adapt".

Stress can also be classified as domestic, social or occupational.

Human Response to Stress

When a person undergoes stress, he may adapt to it if he is resilient. Whenever I see a tall and healthy tree standing firm on its strong foundation, swaying *with* the wind (and not *against* it), withstanding all manner of harsh conditions with resilience, while bearing bountiful fruits and flowers, I always stop to admire it. There can be no better example of how to handle stress and succeed against all odds.

But instead of adapting to adverse conditions, if you resist, you will go into the stage where anxiety develops and if the stressors persist, illness can set in.

Stress and Disease -

All stress is not bad for us. Some amount of stress is needed to keep us keyed up and make us mentally stronger, but if there is continuous or severe stress to which we cannot adapt, illness results. Look at a rubber band — you pull on it and it comes back to normal. But if you keep doing it, over a period of time it loses its elasticity and is not able to come back to its original shape. That is what happens when stress is repeated and persistent.

Stress induced diseases are called psycho (mind) soma (body) or psychosomatic diseases where the body is affected by stress on the mind. There are some early warning symptoms like loss of appetite and sleep, decreased interest in surroundings and appearance, irritability, forgetfulness, new mannerisms, lack of confidence etc., which should warn us that something is wrong and to take remedial action.

Psycho- somatic illnesses can be many — and Diabetes is one of the diseases influenced to a great extent by the state of the mind.

Stress hormones and Diabetes

Blood sugar is increased due to the release of stress hormones like — Adrenaline, nor-adrenaline, cortisol, growth hormone and thyroid hormone.

Simple test to diagnose stress

High alpha amylase levels in saliva indicate that a person is prone to stress related illnesses.

How to handle stress–It is very important for you to be able to handle stress to prevent continuous release of stress hormones that cause increase in your blood sugar; here's how you can do it—

Attitudinal change –

Attitudinal changes are the most effective in reducing stress. Being regular in your work, planning properly, working hard but getting enough relaxation and sleep are important to reduce stress. Also don't get bogged down by *criticism*—Mark Twain the famous American author has said—'no one kicks a dead dog', and "a successful man is one who builds a strong foundation out of bricks thrown at him by others."

Abraham Lincoln has also said—

"If the end brings me out right, then what is said against me does not matter,

And if it brings me out wrong, then ten angels swearing I am right,

Will make no difference"

Also project an effective *outward image* of yourself, since a tidy and unruffled person is more likely to instill confidence in others. A successful person is therefore one, who *like a duck, presents a calm exterior, while paddling furiously underneath.*

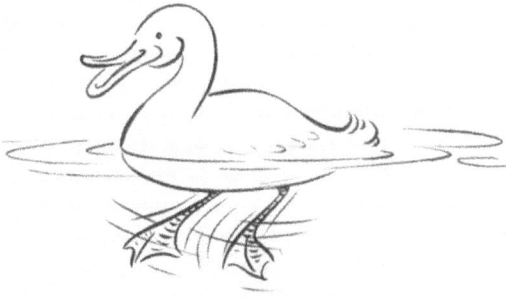

Don't think of people as black or white—Each person should be treated as a different individual, like in a basket of fruits, there are some good ones and some bad, everyone has good and bad traits and we should learn to praise the good ones while tolerating the bad.

Reducing intake of alcohol, tea, coffee, and avoiding smoking are other factors to reduce stress.

Good nutrition, adequate sleep and moderate exercise also help in reducing stress

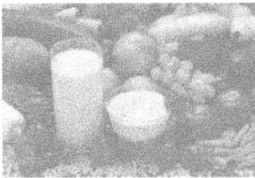

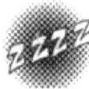

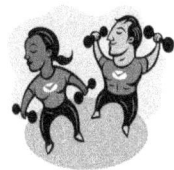

Over the years, many techniques have been developed to combat stress. Let us try to understand some of them since they may help in controlling your blood sugar.

- Improving physical fitness
- Physical relaxation techniques

- Mental relaxation techniques
- Breathing techniques
- Seeking outside help
- Medication

Physical fitness - Improving physical fitness (which can be achieved by walking fifteen kilometers. a week, aerobics or yogic asanas,) is a great de-stressor – 'sound body, is equal to sound mind' – and vice versa.

Physical relaxation – can be achieved by physical training of muscles (by experts), body massage, and shavasana.

Mental relaxation – Mental relaxation can be achieved by shavasana, meditation, listening to soothing music, reading humorous literature, chanting mantras, or saying prayers with beads or rosaries.

Breathing Exercises or Pranayam - Breath is equivalent to 'Prana' or life. When someone gets a brilliant idea, he is 'inspired' and conversely when someone dies, we say he has 'expired'. From this we can gauge the importance of breath. Breath provides us with life giving oxygen to every cell in the body when we breathe in; and removes harmful toxins when we breathe out. It makes us healthier, reduces stress and rejuvenates the Liver, kidneys and Pancreas –the organs that need to function well to keep blood sugar under control.

Seeking outside help –those of you who are stressed should join a social group, laughter club, towel club (each person talks about his sorrows, and everyone empathises), listening to discourses on Bhagvad Gita, Ramayana, Bible or Koran, joining a trekking group etc. to reduce stress.

Psychotherapy - by a trained psychologist, can benefit many of you.

Medications – Medications to reduce stress should be the last resort, and from a psychiatrist. So if stress is the cause of your blood sugars being out of control, do try these measures to bring your Diabetes back under control.

In the next chapter you will learn how to self examine your bodies for complications, and how to self monitor and self inject yourself if you are told to take insulin.

CHAPTER 8

Self-examination and self-injection techniques

Self-examination and Body Care:

You need to take care of your body very meticulously and examine yourselves regularly, as many complications can be prevented from progressing if detected early. You should look out for any infections, discolouration, and loss of sensations on skin. Feet especially need extra care; you need to examine them regularly for any change in look, any swelling, loss of sensation and colour change. Examine the soles for cracks, hard spots, and loss of sensation. Use a reflecting mirror if you find it hard to examine your soles. Don't ignore any coughs, wounds and fevers — they could turn serious. Self examination is extremely important to detect changes early, so that they can be treated and complications prevented.

Self – injection of insulin

Learn everything about insulin injections before you start using them!

Self – injection techniques:

- Before each injection, the hands and the injection site should be clean and top of insulin vial should be wiped with 70% isopropyl alcohol or spirit.

- For all insulin preparations, except rapid- and short-acting insulin and insulin glargine, the vial or pen should be gently rolled in the palms of the hands (not shaken) to re-suspend the insulin.

- An amount of air equal to the dose of insulin required should first be drawn up and injected into the vial to avoid creating a vacuum.

- When mixing rapid- or short-acting insulin with intermediate- or long-acting insulin, the clear rapid- or short-acting insulin should be drawn into the syringe first.

Injection procedure

- Injections should be made into the subcutaneous tissue (just under the skin).

- In thin or averagely built person, lift or grasp a fold of skin between thumb and index finger and inject at 45°or 90°. If you are an obese person, full length injection at 90° is recommended.

With the use of insulin pens, the needle should remain embedded within the skin for 5 sec after complete depression of the plunger to ensure complete delivery of the insulin dose.

Delivery devices

- A compatible syringe having 0-40 U/mL or 100 U/mL should be used for injection (as mentioned on vial).

- The needle used is very fine, of 29 G or 30 G, having either 8 mmol 12.7 mm length suitable for average and obese patients respectively.

- Ideally, a syringe should not be reused but if reuse is desired then after injection recap it and store properly at room temperature in appropriate box.

- Insulin pens are safe, accurate, convenient and most suitable for elderly and handicapped persons. They can be reused and only cartridges need to be replaced. Each cartridge contains 300 U of insulin—so if you are taking 10 U a day, it will last you 30 days.

- Insulin jet injectors inject insulin as a fine stream into the skin. These injectors offer an advantage for patients unable to use syringes or those with needle phobias and more rapid absorption of short-acting insulin. However, the initial cost of these injectors is relatively high, and they may traumatize the skin.

- Others include subcutaneous insulin infusion pumps(see below)

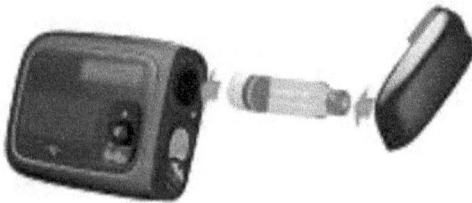

nasal infusion infuser, transdermal infusion, oral infusion etc.The last three are still not popular.

Insulin concentrations: Common available insulin concentrations include 40 IU/mL (U 40), U 100 IU/mL and U500. Care must be taken to ensure that the same concentration is supplied each time a new prescription is made. Mostly U 40 and U 100 insulin syringes are used in India.

Storage of insulin: Insulin must never be frozen. It should be always stored in a cool and dark place. *After opening, an insulin vial should be discarded after 3 months if kept at 2–8°C or after 1 month if kept at room temperature.*

- The best places to inject insulin are the upper arms, the thighs, the buttocks and the abdomen (leave a gap of at least two inches around the navel – (see pictures below).

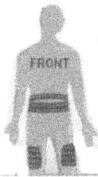

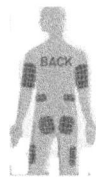

Insulin is absorbed–

- Fastest from the abdomen (stomach)
- A little slower from the arms
- Even slower from the legs
- Slowest from the buttocks

(However, exercising an arm or leg after an injection can increase blood flow and speed insulin absorption from all these areas).

Rotating your injection sites

Injection into the same spot can cause lipohypertrophy (local fat build up),the buildup of fat under the skin, which can slow the absorption of insulin, or lipoatrophy, (the wasting of fat under the skin) which can be unsightly. These are less likely to occur in people using only human insulin).

- It is a good idea to inject your breakfast and lunch bolus doses into the abdomen. Insulin is absorbed fastest when injected into this area. Fast absorption is needed at mealtimes to cover the carbohydrates you are about to eat.

- On the other hand, your supper or bedtime dose of long-acting insulin could be injected into the thigh, buttocks, or upper arm. That's because you want the long-acting insulin to take effect gradually and cover your needs throughout the night.

- Do not inject your lunch bolus dose in the abdomen on Monday and in the thigh on Tuesday. If you have picked the thigh for your evening injection, then continue to use the thigh for all of your evening injections. You can however change from left to right thigh and vice versa.

- If you mix two types of insulin in one shot, you can inject into the abdomen, arm, thigh, or buttocks.

- Work with your doctor and track your blood glucose levels carefully when you begin practicing site rotation. Over time, you and your doctor will learn which injection sites give you the best blood glucose control at different times of day.

- Do not inject close to the belly button. The tissue there is tougher, so the insulin absorption will not be as consistent. For the same reason, do not inject close to moles or scars.

- If you inject in the upper arm, use only the outer back area (where there is most fat). It is hard to pinch the upper arm when you are injecting yourself. Try pressing your upper arm against a wall or door.

- If you inject in the thigh, stay away from the inner thighs. If your thighs rub together when you walk, if might make the injection site sore.

- Do not inject in an area that will be exercised soon. Exercising increases blood flow, which causes long-acting insulin to be absorbed at a rate that's faster than you need.

> Do not inject into an area likely to be exercised soon or absorption will be unusually fast.

- You can reduce injection pain by choosing a needle length and gauge that are right for you.

- Inject in the same area of the body, making sure to move around within that area with each injection, for one or two weeks.

- Then move to another area of your body and repeat the process. Use the same area for at least a week to avoid extreme blood sugar variations.

In the next chapter you will learn how to monitor and track your blood sugar.

CHAPTER 9

Monitoring and tracking

Self-Monitoring of blood glucose (SMBG)Home monitoring

Each of you must have a glucometer and test your sugar at regular intervals

SMBG puts you in a situation in which you can be in control of your own therapy.

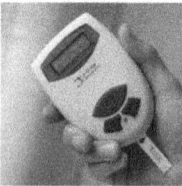

Regular self monitoring of blood glucose, immensely improves control of Diabetes. Every diabetic should self monitor his blood glucose.

Many diabetes self-management programs have demonstrated to help reduce complications. In all of these, SMBG is an integral part of the process. The frequency and type of monitoring in diabetes therapy should be determined on case to case basis by your doctor. SMBG is particularly recommended especially if you have type 2 diabetes and are taking insulin or drugs that cause release of insulin—because it allows you to identify low or high blood glucose. This is especially important in the old and those with long standing Diabetes, who do not experience the warning signs of blood sugar fluctuations.

Choose a glucometer with the help of your doctor that gives a result which is closest to lab reading, does not require coding and there is no loss of strips if inadequate blood is drawn. Glucometers normally give a value 10-20% higher than lab testing for post meal testing. Fasting levels of blood sugar are however almost same for both glucometer and lab readings.

Diabetic card– Every diabetic should carry an identification card stating roughly the following:

- *I am a diabetic*
- *If I faint, give me sugar*
- *My address and phone number is ----*
- *My personal physician's number is ---*
- *I am taking the following medications*

He must also carry his regular drugs and some sugar cubes with him especially if he is on insulin in case his blood sugar drops suddenly.

Diabetes Tracker

Why needed

Every patient must track his Diabetes. At one glance a tracker table gives an idea of the trend of entire profile of the disease, including — examination findings, and the tests performed to assess risk.

DIABETES TRACKER

Why needed

Every patient must track his Diabetes. At one glance a tracker table gives an idea of the trend of entire profile of the disease, including--- examination findings, and the tests performed to assess risk.

Name	Age	Sex	Ht	Wt	BMI	WHR

Parameters	Jan	Feb	Mar	Apr	May	Jun	Jul	Aug	Sep	Oct	Nov	Dec	Target Values	Med
Wt 3 monthly														
Waist circum-ference (Waist height ratio) 3 monthly													<0.5%	
BP 3 monthly													130/80	
FBG 3 monthly													90-130	
PPBG 2 HR 3 monthly													<180	
HbA1c 6 monthly													<7	
LIPIDS Yearly														

Parameters	Jan	Feb	Mar	Apr	May	Jun	Jul	Aug	Sep	Oct	Nov	Dec	Target Values	Med
Chol													<200	
HDL													>40	
LDL													<100	
VLDL													5-40mg/dl	
Apo-B													<130mg/dl	
Tri													<150	
Hb Yearly													>12gms%	
BUN Yearly													<20mg/dl	
Cr Yearly													<1.5mg/dl	
R urine Yearly														
S Pot													3.5-5meq/L	
Micral Mcg/ mg of creat— yearly													N-<30 Micro-31-299 Macro-.300	
24 hr UP Yearly													<150mg/24 hrs	
ECG Yearly														
Fundus Yearly														
Foot Exam 3 monthly														
Stress test Yearly-2 yearly														
Others														

Your doctor will be maintaining this, but those of you who want to be empowered and be real partners in the management of your Diabetes, should maintain one too.

You will want to know about newer methods of treatment. These will be covered in the next chapter.

CHAPTER 10

New drugs and methods of treatment

- Newer insulins like inhaled and oral insulin are in the pipe line. Insulin pumps are available. These can be fixed under the skin by a small surgery and they automatically release the correct amount of insulin in a programmed manner — no need for repeated pricks

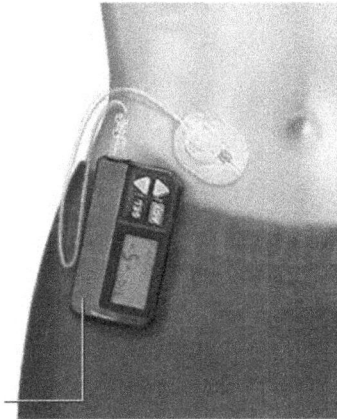

Dose instructions are entered into the small computer on the pump and appropriate amount gets injected into the body in a controlled manner.

- **Berberine**

  Berberine has been used in Chinese medicine for treatment of Diarrhoea. In the eighties it was discovered to have powerful anti Diabetic effect without serious side effects. It is now available in India as an effective drug for Diabetes.

- **DPP-4 inhibitors**

  When we eat, a chemical called incretin is released in the intestines, which causes release of insulin. But action of this chemical is blocked by another chemical called *DPP-4* . It stands to reason that anything that can suppress *DPP-4* will prolong the action of incretin and therefore increase insulin secretion immediately after meals. Two of these drugs –

  Vildagliptin and Sitagliptin are freely available although expensive. Others are in various stages of testing and development.

- **GLP-1 analogs**

  These are incretins that do not get destroyed by DPP4, hence their action is prolonged. Exenatide is intended for once-weekly subcutaneous injection for the treatment of type 2 diabetes. Liraglutide is another drug approved under this category. Both are very expensive and injectable drugs also effective in treating obesity.

- **Saroglitazar**

  A new drug that lowers bad lipids and blood glucose simultaneously

- **Selective sodium glucose co transporter 2 inhibitors (SGLT-I)**

  Kidneys have a big role to play in glucose availability in the body. Each day, they produce 15-55 gms of glucose, use 25-35 gms of glucose for their own energy needs, and filter 180 gms. They also have a role in re-absorbing filtered glucose to maintain optimal blood glucose levels. This process of re -absorption of glucose is through a chemical called SGLT and certain drugs that suppress this chemical, prevent this re-absorption of glucose into the blood. If glucose is not re-absorbed, but allowed to pass out in the urine, blood sugar levels will be lowered. *Dapagliflozin* and *Canagliflozin* are agents in this class that are available.

- **Chloroquine and hydroxyl chloroquine**

  This is an antimalarial drug that lowers blood glucose, and can be used in some patients.

- **New non-injectable Insulins —**

  Buccal — sprayed into mouth and absorbed

  Oral insulin — as tablets

  Transdermal — absorbed through skin

  Inhaled — inhaled through inhaler like asthmatics use. It is called *Afrezza*

- **Stem cell therapy** is also being actively researched. Stem cells are master cells that can turn into any type of cell desired. This is more suitable for type-1 diabetes where pancreatic insulin secreting cells are totally destroyed. Stem cells therapy is also useful in diabetic foot ulcers which are difficult to treat by conventional methods. It is expected that stem cell treatment will increase new vessels in ulcer area so that healing is accelerated.

- **PRP** (platelet rich plasma) therapy also helps in healing of diabetic foot ulcers and is an easier technique than Stem cell therapy.

- **Genetic engineering and pancreatic transplantation** are other exciting prospects.

- **Bionic Pancreas**

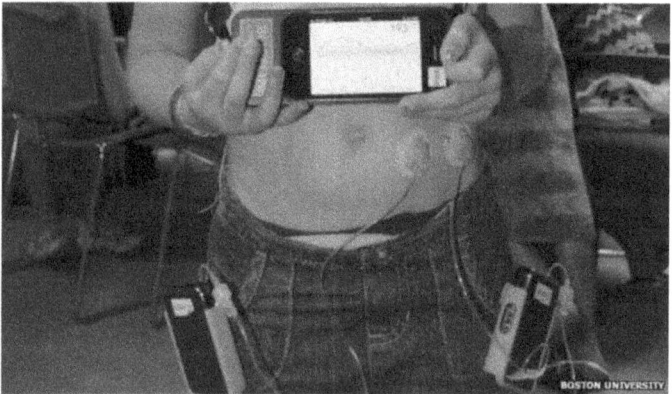

It is like an artificial pancreas — the device uses a smart phone, a continuous blood sugar (glucose) monitor and pumps to automatically deliver the correct quantity of hormones directly into the bloodstream. It mimics a real pancreas by delivering both insulin to lower blood sugar and glucagon to raise it as and when required so patients do not have attacks of either low or high blood sugar.

PART III

COMPLICATIONS OF DIABETES

CHAPTER 11

Overview

If blood sugar remains high for a length of time, it can lead to many complications involving eyes, heart, limbs, brain, and kidneys. Excessive insulin and sugar in the blood leads to changes resulting in high blood pressure, heart attacks, strokes (paralysis), retinopathy (eye involvement), nephropathy (kidney involvement), infections, peripheral angiopathy (involvement of blood vessels) and neuropathy (involvement of nerves).

Like hypertension, diabetes is *a silent killer* if improperly managed. Once the above complications occur, it may be very difficult to reverse unless they are detected early, so it is very important that we prevent them from occurring *by keeping blood glucose under control*

We should be vigilant to detect diabetes and high blood pressure by carrying out regular checkup after 35 years of age , as both these diseases may not produce any symptoms in early stages and may sometimes come to notice for the first time with complications. For example– one patient noticed that his left foot was repeatedly thumping / stamping when he went for walk and then when he got his check up done he was found to have diabetes—he had developed damage to his nerves of the foot even before his diabetes was detected.

> It is important *not to resist taking insulin if it is required to keep diabetes under control.*

How complications occur

Chronic or sustained high blood sugar leads to changes in the inner layer of blood vessels. These changes cause complications all over the body. When larger blood vessels are involved complications that occur are called macro vascular.

Macro vascular complications—examples of large vessel involvement are—

- Cardiovascular disease like ischaemic heart disease or heart attacks,

- Cerebrovascular disease that leads to stroke or paralytic attacks, and

- Peripheral vascular disease that leads to reduced blood supply to the limbs especially legs, leading to severe pains and later bluish discolouration and gangrene (death of the part of limb affected).

When smaller blood vessels are involved, the complications are said to be micro vascular.

Micro vascular complications can be—

- Retinopathy—involvement of eyes

- Nephropathy — involvement of kidneys
- Neuropathy — involvement of nerves

All diabetics must understand that *regularity* is the key in preventing complications.

This includes regularity in observing a restricted diet, medications, blood glucose testing, and check-ups with the doctor, and exercise. If the blood glucose, glycoselated hemoglobin (it gives the average of three months sugar levels) and lipids (bad fats) remain consistently high over a period of time, complications are sure to develop. The commonest complication is either high or low blood sugar which we will discuss in the next chapter.

CHAPTER 12

Hypo and hyper glycaemia

Hypoglycemia — low blood sugar

You should learn the symptoms of *hypoglycemia* (low blood sugar) and to deal with it quickly when it occurs since you are going to suffer from this problem often, especially if you are on insulin or drugs that act by secreting insulin. These symptoms may be —

- Giddiness
- Palpitations
- Sweating
- Headache
- Hunger
- Disturbed sleep

In the elderly diabetic, some of *these warning symptoms may be blunted due to involvement of their autonomic nervous system,* so they should maintain regularity in checkups meals and exercise , and monitor regularly, as any irregularity can cause low blood sugar which may not be recognized and lead to loss of consciousness and even coma.

Management of hypoglycemia — If you have any of these symptoms, first call for help — and then test your blood glucose. If it is above 80 mgs %–just eat something non sweet. But if below – eat a banana, or a few spoons of sugar and follow up with a meal. Monitor your sugar frequently till it comes to at least 120mg, and if it does not — go to a hospital or contact your doctor — do not panic!

Hyperglycaemia — high blood sugar

As is the case with low blood sugar , a diabetic may also have such occasions when his blood sugar rises to very high level on account of some alteration in diet exercise , work schedule , hence it is very important to recognize early signs of high blood sugar which include —

- Increased thirst.
- Headaches.
- Dryness of mouth
- Difficulty concentrating.
- Blurred vision, heaviness in eyes.
- Frequent urination.
- Disturbed sleep
- Fatigue (weak, tired feeling)
- Weight loss.

If you have any of these symptoms check your blood sugar and if high, inform your doctor by SMS, E-mail or phone to help you take corrective action.

CHAPTER 13

Neuropathy and musculo skeletal complications

Nerves, muscles, bones and joints are also commonly involved if your blood sugar remains out of control for long. We will discuss these in this chapter.

Neuropathy

Diabetes can affect the nerves in your body and depending on the nerves affected it is called *autonomic neuropathy* leading to attacks of giddiness or diarrhoea, *motor neuropathy* leading to weakness of muscles resulting in deformities, and *sensory neuropathy* leading to tingling numbness and loss of sensation.

When the nerves of the foot are affected, we call it a *neuropathic foot.*

Foot drop, or experiencing a thud while walking, can be a warning sign of Diabetes. You may also get a feeling of walking on cotton wool. But the commonest complaint is of burning feet if you have neuropathy.

When both the arteries and the nerves are affected, it is called *'Neuro-ischaemic foot'.*

Because of loss of sensation, chances of injury are more since you may be unaware of pain and heat. Neuropathy also leads to deformity of the foot, because the muscles are also affected. This deformity additionally makes you prone to injury.

Musculoskeletal Complications of Diabetes Mellitus

Muscles, bones and skeleton get affected in Diabetes because of many reasons. There is glycoselation of proteins — that is, sugar in the blood combines with proteins. This glycoselation of proteins leads to micro vascular changes (involvement of small blood vessels), damage of blood vessels and nerves, this leads to inflammation, swelling and formation of fibrous (thick, non elastic) bands.

Diabetic cheiroarthropathy, is a condition where there is stiffness of the hand or limitation in movement at joints of hands.

Flexor tenosynovitis (or trigger finger) is a condition where a joint of the finger gets 'locked' and cannot be straightened because of pain

Dupuytren's contracture is due to involvement of fascia (tissue) in the palm of the hand and as the name suggests, the fingers are 'contracted' or pulled and painful.

Carpal tunnel syndrome (CTS) is due to entrapment of median nerve under the tunnel in the front of the wrist, through which blood vessels, nerves and tendon attachment of muscles, pass from forearm to hand.

The pain may awaken patients from sleep and is aggravated by movement involving wrist such as holding a newspaper or book, typing, driving, or using a knife and fork.

Frozen Shoulder

Frozen shoulder affects 10-20 percent of people with diabetes according to the American Academy of Orthopaedic Surgeons. Women are more likely to develop frozen shoulder than men and it occurs mostly in those between the ages of 40 and 60. Frozen shoulder syndrome, or adhesive capsulitis, occurs when ligaments (that attach one bone to another) around the shoulder joint swell and stiffen to such an extent that normal healing doesn't take place. This makes it difficult to move the shoulder, making everyday activities such as getting dressed or reaching for a cup from a shelf painful. As the condition progresses, the stiffness may continue to the point where range of motion can be severely limited, and shoulder gets 'frozen' in one position.

Frozen shoulder has three stages:

1. **Freezing** — Pain slowly becomes worse until range of motion is lost. (Lasts 6 weeks to 9 months)

2. **Frozen** — Pain improves, but the shoulder is still stiff. (Lasts 4 to 6 months)

3. **Thawing** — Ability to move the shoulder improves until normal or close to normal. (Lasts 6 months to 2 years)

Early symptoms of frozen shoulder

- A feeling of pain and tightness in the shoulder area.

- A feeling of tightness especially when putting the arm up and back, as you would do it you were throwing a ball over arm.

- Pain on the back of the wrist. (This specifically relates to frozen shoulder caused by subscapularis trigger points.)

- As time goes on, the symptoms will worsen although the pain may be reduced.

Treatments for frozen shoulder

- Anti-inflammatory drugs and pain killers like aspirin and ibuprofen.

- Exercises and stretching at home — keep moving and stretching the shoulder

- Keep two pillows — one under head and the other between elbow and body of affected hand

- Always try to keep arm away from body while sitting for long

- Massage with hot oil

- Local heat

- Physiotherapy by a trained person
- NAT (Niel Asher Technique)

  Research from Cambridge University Hospitals looked at the Niel Asher Technique (NAT) – a method involving the manipulation of muscle tissues and joints, applying pressure and stretching –Improvement was 52% as compared to 24%. – Consult your Physiotherapist.

- Acupuncture works by pinpointing certain pressure points on the body, thereby reducing inflammation. – but do consult an accredited acupuncturist.

- Manipulation of joint under the effect of anaesthesia

- Injecting steroid injection locally

- Corrective surgery

Calcific periarthritis of the shoulder is also seen in diabetes. Shoulder x-rays show calcium deposits outside the joint, in the area of the rotator cuff tendons.

Reflex sympathetic dystrophy also known as "shoulder-hand syndrome," is seen in diabetic patients. It may be associated with frozen shoulder (with or without calcific periarthritis).

Patients may complain of pain from shoulder to hand in the affected limb. There may be swelling, skin changes (changes in hair growth, shiny skin, color and temperature changes), and increased sensitivity to temperature and touch. Patchy osteoporosis or thinning of bones is also often seen. Early treatment is important. Drugs that reduce inflammation, pain reducing drugs, and corticosteroids can be used along with physio therapy. Sometimes sympathetic nerve block injections may be required — that numb the nerves that sense pain.

Diabetic osteoarthropathy(Charcot or neuropathic arthropathy) is a condition affecting the feet. Due to loss of sensation and repeated minor injuries, there is destruction of the joint.

Treatment involves both splinting/bracing/partial cast to protect the area from weight bearing and good sugar control. Sometimes a total cast may be required which has to be changed frequently.

Diabetic muscle infarction (death of muscle) is a rare condition. There is a sudden onset of pain and swelling over days to weeks in the affected muscles (usually the thigh or calf).

Treatment consists of rest and pain killers. Gentle routine daily activities can be carried out. This condition tends to resolve over a period of weeks to months in most cases.

Diffuse idiopathic skeletal hyperostosis (DISH)– there is calcification and stiffness of spinal ligaments that connect the spinal vertebra to each other.

You may feel stiffness in the neck and back with decreased range of motion. Pain is generally not a prominent symptom. Treatment consists of physiotherapy and drugs that reduce inflammation and pain.

Management of Diabetic complications of musculo-skeleton

- Control blood glucose
- NSAIDS(anti inflammatory drugs)
- Exercises
- Local steroid injection
- Manipulation and physiotherapy
- Massage by a qualified masseur, or physiotherapist.
- Heat
- Surgery

In the next chapter we discuss in detail the complications that can occur in the feet, and how to care for them.

CHAPTER 14

DIABETIC FOOT/FOOT CARE IN DIABETES

Diabetes can affect the feet due to neuropathy (affecting nerves) leading to loss of sensation, angiopathy (affecting blood vessels) leading to less blood supply to feet, and infections and non healing wounds that become worse because of loss of sensation and reduced blood supply. If the non healing wound persists, it can lead to gangrene or death of the part and even amputation or the need to cut off part of the foot or leg to prevent the spread of gangrene.

Feet are one of the most important but neglected parts of our body.

Consider the functions they perform -

- They bear the whole load of our body

- They help us in locomotion (movement)

- They are indispensable while riding or driving a vehicle

- Not for nothing do *FEET* rhyme with FEAT. If you take good care of your feet, you can perform any feat that a non-diabetic can, and leave your "footprints, on the sands of time".

Heels are also very important because if you don't walk enough or wear wrong shoes (tight, narrow, and high heels), there may be growth of the anklebone called 'calcaneal spur' which again may have to be operated on.

Your legs are also responsible for pumping blood back to the heart. That is why calves are also called 'peripheral heart'. If the calf muscles are weak, or there is fat deposition in the muscles, this pumping action is impaired and blood will collect in the ankles leading to swelling. This also leads to break down of the "one-way valves" which are present *in the veins* of the legs. As we know, veins carry blood back to heart and lungs for purification. Valves in the veins prevent the impure blood from flowing back downwards. But if they are damaged, the blood does not go up but stagnates in the legs. This further increases the swelling and since the veins cannot bear the load of the extra blood in them, they become twisted and tortuous. This is called ' varicose veins '(blue and twisted veins)

Arteries (they are the blood vessels that carry purified blood from the heart to the rest of the body) and nerves (they recognize sensations — pain, temperature, pressure etc) are also important in the legs. If the arteries are blocked, blood supply to the part of the limb beyond the block, is impaired and the tissues may die, and if the nerves are affected, there may be tingling, numbness and loss of sensation, which may make us unaware of heat, cold or pain, leading to ulcers.

We care for our hands and face but since feet are mostly invisible, we don't give them much thought. Once in a while, you might scrub them clean and haphazardly cut the toenails - that is all. But foot care is extremely important. You must inspect your feet regularly, wash and scrub them daily, look for corns and callosities (tough skin) and if they are present, attend to them immediately under the care of a qualified doctor/ foot specialist. Do not try home surgery. Cracked heels are not only cosmetically ugly, but can become quite painful. Learning to trim your toenails correctly is also important. Toenails should be cut square and the margins should not be cut, or the nails may grow inwards into the skin. This "in-growing" of toenails is painful and will need surgery to correct it. Healing is always a slow process in a diabetic.

Guidelines for foot care in Diabetes

Shoes and socks–

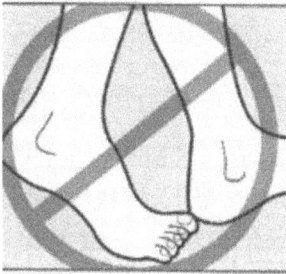

Do not walk barefoot even at home

Always protect your feet by wearing shoes or hard-soled slippers or footwear, or at least thick cotton socks;

- Avoid shoes with high heels and pointed toes; Avoid shoes that expose your toes or heels (such as open-toed shoes or sandals). These types of shoes increase your risk for injury and potential infections; Try on new footwear with the type of socks you usually wear; Do not wear new shoes for more than an hour at a time; Wear good quality leather or canvas shoes with square or rounded toes, and good depth, low heels and Velcro, lace or buckles for comfortable and secure fitting;

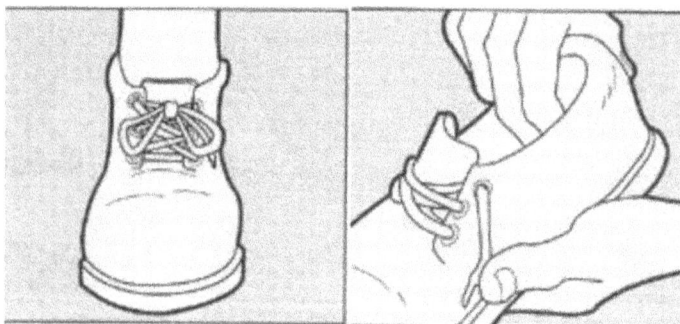

- Inspect your shoes daily for pebbles, cracks, or anything that can hurt your feet. Look and feel inside your shoes); Make sure your shoes fit properly. If you have neuropathy (nerve damage), you may not notice that your shoes are too tight;

- Change your socks daily;

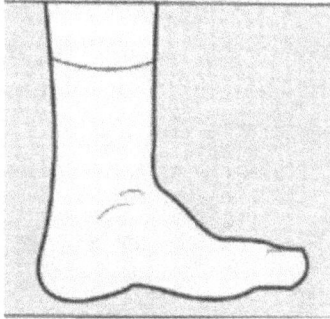

Before putting them on make sure there are no foreign objects or rough areas. Avoid tight socks, with tight elastic; Wear natural-fiber socks (cotton, wool, or a cotton-wool blend

- If you get a blister or sore from your shoes, do not "burst" it. Apply a bandage and wear a different pair of shoes; If ulcers have already developed or some potential points are there where ulcers can develop, then special padded insoles can be used to protect these points; Special footwear can also be designed to serve individual needs. These will help in healing of existing ulcers and prevent new ones.

Buy shoes in the evening, because size of feet is maximum in the evening

Do not wear acupressure slippers or toe strap slippers

***Cleaning*-**Clean feet with lukewarm water and soap twice daily then wipe dry-Use mild soaps; Pat your skin dry; do not rub; Thoroughly dry your feet especially between toes, ; After washing, use lotion on your feet to prevent cracking. Do not put lotion between your toes.

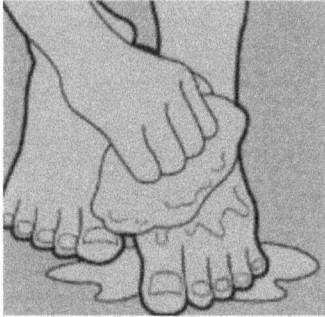

***Inspection*-**Inspect feet daily for wounds, blisters &temperature changes (hot or cold);

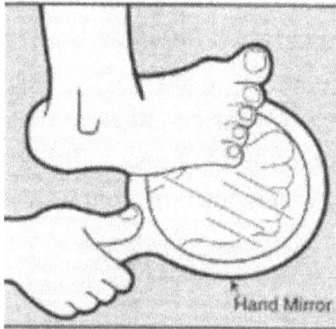

Check the tops and bottoms of your feet; Have someone else look at your feet if you cannot see them or use a mirror or magnifying glass. Check for dry, cracked skin; Look for blisters, cuts, scratches, or other sores; Check for redness, increased warmth, or tenderness when touching any area of your feet; Check for ingrown toenails, corns, and calluses. Dry feet after bath especially between toes

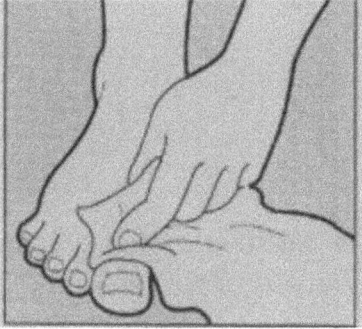

Applications–Do not apply hot or cold fomentation, heating pads, strong or irritant ointments. If the skin is dry, special moisturizing creams can be used but not between toes. Do not do vigorous maalish/massage.

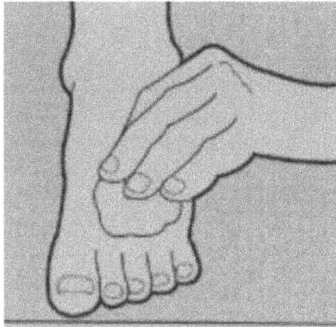

Nails — Cut your toe nails regularly and cut square (not rounded). Avoid cutting into the corners of nails and the best time to do this is just after a bath, when they are soft. After cutting them, smooth them with a nail file;

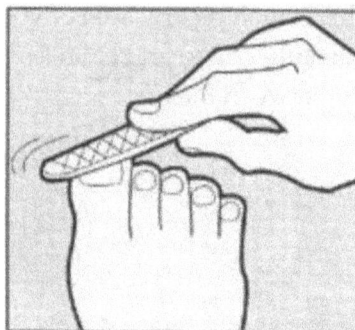

you may want a podiatrist (foot doctor) to cut your toenails if they have ingrown into your skin at the sides.

There are several precautions that you need to observe while going to the temple— — Try to wear thick socks when you go to a temple. Avoid walking on hot or rough floors in temples. Do not take off your footwear on the road/ path to the temple.

Wear thick socks inside a temple. Avoid walking on hot or rough floors inside the temple. Do not take off your foot wear on the road /path leading to temple *especially in summer—you may suffer injury or burns*

*Exercise-*Walking is the safest exercise for the feet; Walk in comfortable shoes; Do not exercise when you have open sores on your feet. Do not walk too fast or take long strides. Shorter walks, more frequent and small steps are advised especially for those with neuropathic problems. Do not stand for long. Standing puts whole body weight on feet.

Management of burning feet–your doctor will give you B-12, ALA supplements and other drugs. You can apply a moisturizer and cream containing capsaicin every night.

Prevention of diabetic foot–to prevent diabetic foot, tight blood glucose control has to be maintained. Body weight, blood pressure, and lipids should also be controlled. You must completely STOP smoking. Diabetes leads to changes in blood vessels, and smoking adds to it. The combination can be deadly. So you have no choice but to stop unless you want to lose your feet or even your legs.

Do not sit cross-legged for long.

Do not stand on hot road or surface.

Never do home surgery for corns, thorns and boils.

Do not soak your feet in hot or ice-cold water.

Exercises for Feet

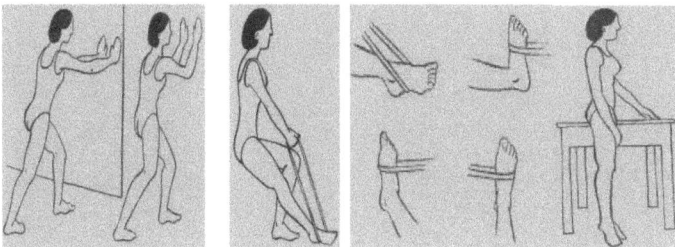

1) Push against the wall	2)Pull with rope — up, down, side to side	3)Stand on toes at full stretch with hand on table for support

4)Keep some marbles on a mat and pick up with toes.

You must have a session with your doctor/diabetic educator on foot care to learn everything scientifically.

CHAPTER 15

EYE COMPLICATIONS IN DIABETES

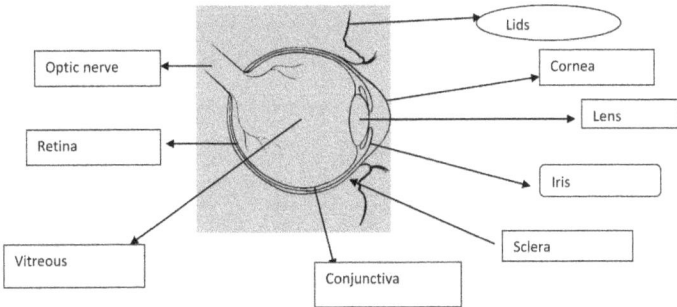

Lids
Cornea
Lens
Iris
Sclera
Conjunctiva
Optic nerve
Retina
Vitreous

EYE COMPLICATIONS IN DIABETES CAN BE—

- Diabetic Retinopathy(screen or retina behind eyes)
- Diabetic cataract
- Glaucoma due to diabetes
- Diabetic neuropathy (nerves of eyes)
- Infections in eye
- Vascular blocks and ischemia (blood vessels of eyes)

DIABETIC RETINOPATHY

Diabetic retinopathy is a condition where the screen at the back of the eye called retina gets affected, leading to bleeding, cotton wool like spots, central swelling, disturbance of vision, and later even blindness.

Some facts about Diabetic retinopathy

It is the leading cause of blindness in diabetics aged 20-74 years. Nearly all Type 1 and 75% of Type 2 diabetes patients will develop retinopathy after 15 year duration of diabetes.

But the encouraging news is that — even a 1% reduction in HbA1c, reduces the risk of retinopathy by 40%.

And a 10 mm Hg reduction in systolic blood pressure decreases the risk of retinopathy progression by 35%. This should keep you motivated to maintain a good control of your blood sugar at all times.

The prevalence and severity of Diabetic retinopathy is higher in south east Asians than in Whites.

Dyslipidaemia (disturbed fats), cataract surgery, reduced physical activity, low socioeconomic status, increased body mass index and consumption of alcohol are some other risk factors that increase the incidence of Diabetic Retinopathy. Table below shows recommendations of American academy of Ophthalmology about frequency of eye examination for a diabetic

Recommendations of American Academy of Ophthalmology,

	Type -1	Type-2	GDM
Recommended first eye examination	Within 5 years after diagnosis	At time of diagnosis of diabetes	Prior to conception and during first trimester
Minimal routine follow-up	yearly	Two yearly till DR is detected, then yearly	Depending on previous results — every trimester

Treatment of Diabetic retinopathy

Laser treatment

In this laser waves are used to seal or destroy (photocoagulate) abnormal leaking blood vessels in retina which develop in diabetic retinopathy .

Either the whole retina, or only central portion is subjected to it.

Surgery

Vitreous lies in front of the retina and the space between retina and vitreous develops thick bands pulling and 'detaching' the retina in those with persistently high blood sugar. To prevent this detachment, eye surgeons remove the vitreous. This is called vitrectomy.

Other treatment options for Diabetic retinopathy – (you can discuss with your eye doctor)

- Vascular endothelial growth factor (VEGF) inhibitors
- Protein kinase C inhibitor
- Steroids
- Somatostatin
- Interferon alpha 2a
- Statins: 3-hydroxy-3-methyl-glutaryl coenzyme A reductase Inhibitors
- Hyperbaric Oxygen

DIABETIC CATARACT

High blood glucose and long duration of Diabetes leads to early and more rapid development of cataract (lens becomes opaque) . The risk of cataract is 2–4 times greater in diabetics than in non-diabetics and may be 15–25 times greater in diabetics under 40 years old with women developing cataracts slightly more than men. Snowflake cataract is a type of cataract seen in Type I Diabetes.

Cataracts may be reversible in young diabetics with improvement in glucose control.

GLAUCOMA

Glaucoma is increase in pressure inside the eyes, that can even lead to loss of vision. In Diabetics, it occurs due to proliferation of new vessels.

- The risk of glaucoma has been reported to be 1.6–4.7 times in diabetics

- Sealing or destroying new vessels (pan retinal photo-coagulation by laser) is the standard option to prevent development of glaucoma, as proliferation of new vessels is the cause of glaucoma in diabetes.

DIABETIC NEUROPATHY(nerves of the eye)

Diabetic neuropathy is involvement of the nerves related to the eyes, leading to paralysis of muscles around that help in moving our eyeballs. It is seen in 25–30% of patients aged 45 years and older who develop acute muscle paralysis around the eyes. It can also lead to dryness of eyes and even ulcer formation. When the main nerve in the eye called *optic nerve* (that carries signals to the brain helping us to see things) is affected, it is called anterior ischemic optic neuropathy (AION), This Is a dangerous complication and can lead to sudden blindness in a diabetic.

INFECTIONS IN EYES

When Diabetes remains uncontrolled, and the blood glucose is high, eyes can get infected like the rest of the body, which can even lead to blindness

Rhino cerebral mucormycosis is a fungal infection that can spread to the brain through the nose and can be fatal.

VASCULAR BLOCKS AND ISCHEMIA

Diabetes can cause blocks inside blood vessels in the eyes—this can be in arteries, veins or smaller blood vessels called arterioles.

Retinal artery occlusion (RAO) is a condition similar to emboli (tiny blocks that arise from distant parts of the body and reach the blood vessels in the eyes).

Patient experiences a sudden, unilateral, painless loss of vision or a visual defect in peripheral vision when this occurs.

CHAPTER 16

KIDNEY COMPLICATIONS IN DIABETES
(Diabetic nephropathy)

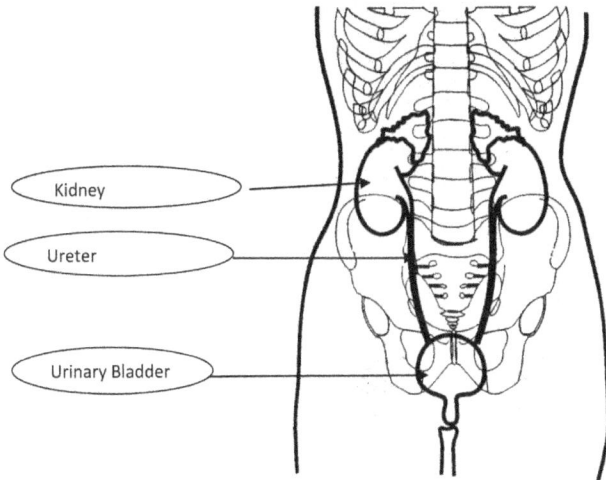

Diabetic nephropathy is a progressive kidney disease seen in those patients with long standing uncontrolled Diabetes and caused by angiopathy (involvement of the blood vessels inside it. Small vessels are particularly involved—that is why it is called a 'micro'vascular complication). It is one of the leading causes of ESRD (end stage renal disease) needing Dialysis and kidney transplantation. *Remember, it is totally preventable if you maintain strict blood glucose control.* Once the kidneys fail, the function of removing toxins from the body is by a process called Dialysis which has to be continued at regular intervals life-long. The only solution at this stage is to transplant a kidney from a donor. Getting a matching donor may not be easy and the cost can be prohibitive — so 'CONTROL and PREVENTION' are the keys at your command to be used to prevent Diabetic nephropathy. Changes in blood vessels, leads to hardening and loss of function of the basic unit of the kidney called glomerulus. Once the kidney structure hardens, its function fails, there is loss of protein in the urine, leading to foamy urine, and fluid retention manifesting as swelling or oedema. It begins with puffiness around the eyes, especially in the morning, later in the legs and all over the body, leading to weight gain. Because of narrowing of blood vessels inside the kidneys, there is release of a chemical called Renin—that leads to progressive increase in blood pressure. And because kidney functions are disturbed, there is accumulation of toxins like urea and creatinine in the blood. Other symptoms are poor appetite, nausea, vomiting, weakness, and hiccups.

How Diabetic nephropathy occurs—the whole process explained

When there is too much sugar in the blood, all of it cannot be reabsorbed by the kidneys like it normally happens. The extra sugar is passed out in the urine, raising its osmotic pressure, and causing more water to be drawn out along with it, thus, increasing the excreted urine volume. The increased volume also dilutes the sodium chloride in the urine, signaling the kidneys to release a chemical called renin, that causes narrowing of blood vessels. This chemical is also secreted when there is fall in blood pressure or narrowing of blood vessels. Renin leads to high blood pressure; Narrowing of blood vessels also leads to hardening and death of tissues in the kidneys. In the initial stages there is a little loss of albumin due to changes in the inner lining of blood vessels and increased permeability of the glomerulus in the urine called microalbuminuria. Later there is more loss of albumin, called macro albuminuria, followed by increase in toxins like urea and creatinine in blood, signaling kidney failure.

Lab tests

There is protein in the urine called albumin which initially is at the microscopic level.

> Microalbumin in the urine is a Red flag . It is a cry of the kidney requesting you to control blood sugar at least now if you have been complacent before .

When it increases, it becomes obvious in the routine examination of urine. It is therefore very important to check microscopic albumin in urine regularly to detect and possibly reverse it at an early stage so that you do not progress to the next stage and possibly end stage kidney failure.

- Normal albuminuria: urinary albumin excretion <30 mg/24h

- Microalbuminuria: urinary albumin excretion in the range of 30–299 mg/24h

- Clinical (overt) albuminuria: urinary albumin excretion ≥300 mg/24h.

Microalbuminuria can be tested by doing a spot urine examination or collecting a 24 hour sample to assess amount of protein being lost per day.

Later on the blood toxins like urea and serum creatinine also rise and this indicates beginning of end stage kidney disease

Kidney biopsy can confirm the diagnosis, although normally it is not required since the diagnosis is obvious.

CKD—chronic kidney disease—correlation between Glomerular filtration rate (GFR) which is another test that can be performed, and stage of kidney failure—

CKD Stage	eGFR level (mL/min/1.73 m²)
Stage 1	≥ 90
Stage 2	60 – 89
Stage 3	30 – 59
Stage 4	15 – 29
Stage 5	< 15

As you can see, the GFR progressively reduces as the chronic kidney disease progresses. From the chart below, you can understand where you are placed with respect to kidney involvement—

Development of Diabetic Nephropathy[3]

Stage	Designation	Characteristics	Structural Changes	Glomerular Filtration Rate mL/ min 1.73 m^2	Blood Pressure mm Hg
I	Hyperfunction	Hyperfiltration	Glomerular hypertrophy	>150	Normal
II	Normoalbuminuria	Normal albumin loss	Basement membrane thickening	150	Normal
III	Incipient diabetic nephropathy (microalbuminuria)	Increased albumin loss	Albumin loss correlates with structural damage and hypertrophy of remaining glomeruli	125	Increased
IV	Overt diabetic nephropathy	Clinical proteinuria	Advanced structural damage	<100	Hypertension
V	Uremia-blood urea and creatinine increased	Kidney failure	Glomerular closure	0-10	High

Some facts about Diabetic nephropathy

- Nephropathy has been reported to occur in 20-40% of patients with diabetes and is the single leading cause of ESRD (end stage renal disease), accounting for >40% of patients requiring renal transplantation each year in developed countries.

- The incidence of diabetic nephropathy is sharply increasing in the developing world, with the Asia-Pacific region being the most severely affected. Nearly 30% of chronic renal failures in India are due to diabetic nephropathy.

- Nephropathy develops in 50% of Diabetics after 20 years of diagnosis

- 15% already are in ESRD at the time of diagnosis of Diabetes

- Genetic susceptibility, race/ethnicity, poor sugar control and hypertension are the major predisposing factors of diabetic nephropathy.

- Other risk factors include *high protein intake, high lipid levels and smoking*

How to avoid kidney damage

As I have repeatedly stressed, blood-glucose levels should be closely monitored and controlled. This may slow the progression of kidney damage, especially in the very early ("microalbuminuria") stages when the damage can be reversed.

One thing to note—as kidney damage worsens, less insulin is thrown out by the kidneys--so more insulin is available. Therefore if your insulin requirement suddenly comes down, without apparent reason—don't celebrate! It may signal kidney damage.

Besides controlling blood sugar, blood pressure should also be aggressively controlled, since it can independently damage the kidneys. Keeping blood lipids, and weight under control is also important and regular physical activity will control blood pressure, blood glucose and kidney damage. Protein intake should be restricted to 0.8 gm/Kg body weight /day and *smoking should be stopped.*

Patients with diabetic nephropathy should avoid taking the following drugs:

- Contrast agents containing iodine — used for some x-rays and CT Scans.

- Commonly used non-steroidal anti-inflammatory drugs (NSAIDs) like ibuprofen and naproxen, or COX-2 inhibitors like celecoxib, because they may injure the weakened kidney — ask your doctor. In fact while I am about it —

Let me caution those of you that regularly consume pain killers. This is an absolute NO in Diabetes

Urinary tract and other infections are common and can be treated with appropriate antibiotics.

Dialysis may be necessary once end-stage renal disease develops. At this stage, a kidney transplantation can also be considered. Another option for type 1 diabetes patients is a combined kidney-pancreas transplant. But these are not ideal options. Remember your goal is to avoid reaching this stage by controlling blood glucose, blood pressure and bad fats.

C-peptide, a by-product of insulin production, may provide new hope for patients suffering from diabetic kidney involvement.

High homocysteine levels in the blood increase its stickiness and can damage the kidneys. This is commonly due to low folic acid (a type of vitamin). You can correct this by taking folic acid supplements and a high folate diet – tomatoes, green beans, spinach, lady's finger, lentil and black-eyed peas.

Management of ESRD (End stage renal disease)

Kidneys are responsible for removing toxins from the body. When their function is lost, Dialysis is used to remove the toxins – blood is taken out, toxins removed and then the blood is reintroduced into the body. Let me explain how this is done –

Dialysis Haemodialysis and peritoneal dialysis are the two types of dialysis.

HAEMODIALYSIS

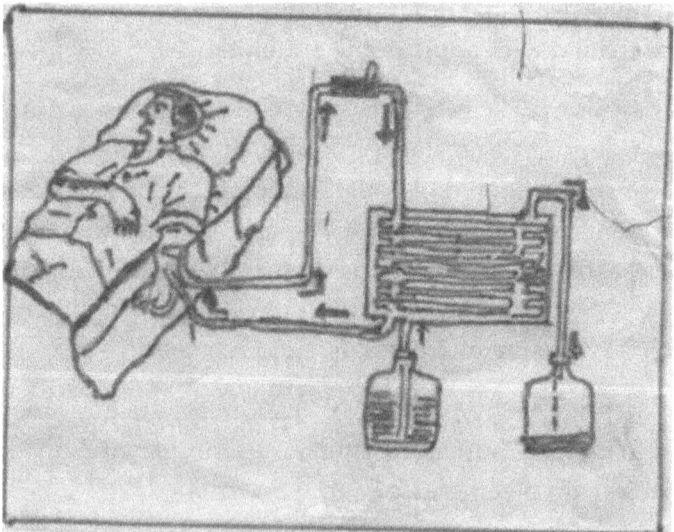

The first step in haemodialysis is to create a connection between an artery and vein in your wrist or hand (AV fistula). This is to make the blood vessel used to transfer blood to and from the body, larger and stronger. The procedure is carried out by a small surgery about six weeks before the beginning of Dialysis sessions to give enough time for healing.

The actual procedure

The actual procedure of dialysis lasts about 4 hours, and most people will require three such sessions a week. Two thin needles are inserted into the AV fistula and taped in place. One needle will be used to remove blood very slowly — 40-50 ml at a time, and transfer it to a machine that contains a series of semi-permeable membranes that filter out toxins, thus acting like the kidneys. A Fluid called Dialysate is then pumped into the artificial kidneys to receive the toxins that are filtered out. The contaminated liquid is pumped out and the cleaned blood is transferred back into your body through the second needle. The same cycle is repeated till all the blood is purified. Usually there are no problems, but some people may experience nausea, dizziness and muscle cramps during the procedure. After the dialysis session, the needles are removed and a plaster is applied to prevent bleeding.

Hemodialysis and fluid intake

Normally, healthy kidneys constantly remove excess fluid from the body. But this does not happen when the kidneys have failed. During the haemodialysis process, two to three days' worth of fluid is removed over the course of four hours. If you drink too much water or fluids, the dialyser will be unable to remove all of the fluid and excess will build up in your blood, tissues and lungs. This can be serious and lead to:

- Breathing difficulties

- High blood pressure

- Coronary heart disease

  The amount of fluid you are allowed to drink will depend on your size and weight. Most people are only allowed to drink 1,000-1,500ml (two to three pints) of fluid a day.

  You will also need to avoid eating foods that have a high fluid content —

- Soups

- Juices

- Tomatoes, oranges, water melon

Chewing gum or sucking an ice cube may help alleviate your symptoms of thirst.

Hemodialysis and diet

As well as removing waste products, your kidneys help regulate the amount of salts and minerals in your body, including:

- sodium

- potassium

- phosphorus

Excess levels of any of these minerals in kidney failure can be dangerous and lead to:

- Fits
- Coma
- Thinning of the bones
- An irregular heart beat
- And even sudden death

You will therefore have to avoid foods rich in sodium, potassium and phosphorus

Foods high in salt (sodium) include:

- Ready-to-eat meals from restaurants
- Preserved and packaged foods
- Bacon
- Ham
- Smoked fish
- Commercial butter
- Cheese

Foods high in potassium include:

- Bananas
- Baked potatoes
- Oranges
- Chocolate

Foods high in phosphorus include:

- Dairy products, such as cheese

- Yoghurt

- Baked beans

- Lentils

- Sardines — a type of fish

- Bran cereals

  The second type of Dialysis is Peritoneal Dialysis —

PERITONEAL DIALYSIS

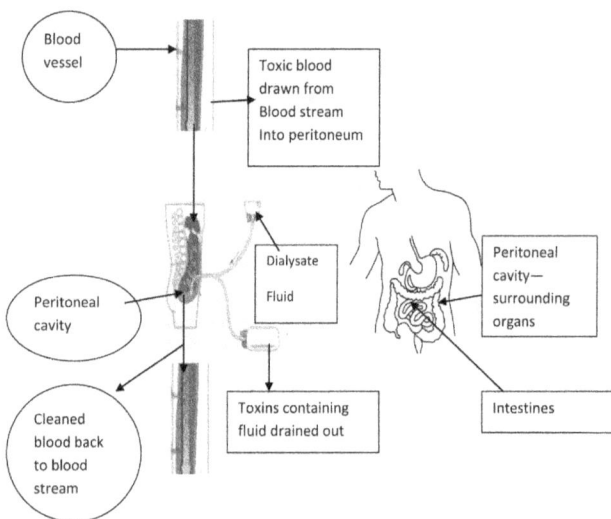

Peritoneum is a lining inside your abdomen, consisting of two layers, between which is a fluid called peritoneal fluid. This fluid is used as an artificial kidney for Dialysis. To create an access point, an incision is made in your abdomen, usually just below your belly button. A piece of equipment called a Tenckhoff catheter is then inserted into the incision .A Tenckhoff catheter is a thin piece of tube, about 10cm (four inches) long The dialysate fluid is passed through this catheter and into the peritoneal cavity. The Peritoneal cavity also receives blood containing toxins from the blood stream. The Dialysate fluid draws out toxins from the blood and the contaminated fluid is drained out. The Tenckhoff catheter is permanently attached to your abdomen. After a dialysis session is complete, the end of the catheter is sealed.

The fluid introduced can be as much as 2.5 litres, and medication can also be added to the fluid immediately before infusion.

Types of peritoneal dialysis

There are two main types of peritoneal dialysis. They are:

- Continuous ambulatory peritoneal dialysis (CAPD) – where your blood is filtered several times during the day

- Automated peritoneal dialysis (APD) – where a machine filters your blood during the night as you sleep

Continuous ambulatory peritoneal dialysis

CAPD can be carried out at home without any help, once everything is in place, and you are trained.

The equipment used to carry out CAPD consists of–

- A bag containing the dialysate fluid

- An empty bag used to collect waste products

- A series of tubing and clips used to secure both bags to the catheter

- A wheeled stand that you can hang both bags from

An exchange begins by draining the old fluid into the waste bag. The new fluid is then drained into your peritoneal cavity. The process is painless and takes about 30-40 minutes to complete.

The new fluid is left in the peritoneal cavity for a number of hours. As blood passes through the peritoneum, special chemicals in the dialysate fluid draw out waste products and excess fluid from the blood into the fluid. The cleaned fluid goes back into the circulation.

After the set number of hours has passed, you will begin the process again, exchanging the old fluid for the new fluid. Most people who use CAPD require four exchanges a day.

You will be fully trained on how to carry out both types of draining, and will be given detailed instructions about how to keep all of the equipment clean to prevent infection. The only problem is that the process is cumbersome and catheter is always in place.

Automated peritoneal dialysis (APD)

Automated peritoneal dialysis (APD) works on the same principles as CAPD, except that a machine is used to control the drainage of fluid. You fill the APD machine with fluid before you go to bed. As you sleep, the machine automatically performs a number of exchanges.

You will usually need to be attached to the APD machine for 8-10 hours. You will then usually have one last fill of fluid that is kept in your cavity all day before it is drained away the following evening. During the night, an exchange can be temporarily interrupted if, for example, you need to go to the toilet. It is usually safe to miss one night's worth of exchanges as long as you resume treatment within 24 hours.

KIDNEY TRANSPLANTATION

Kidney transplantation is the only treatment option that can give a permanent cure to chronic renal failure. A matching donor kidney from a live donor/ or brain dead donor is transplanted into the patient.

Procedure

The donor kidney obtained from either a live or brain-dead donor is transplanted by joining to an artery (Aorta) and vein (Inferior vena cava) much lower than in the original — see picture below. The ureter, of the new kidney, (ureter connects the kidney to the bladder) is fixed into the urinary bladder. The damaged kidneys are not removed. Surgery is performed by cutting open the abdomen, laparoscopically, with small incisions, or even through vagina in women — who have undergone removal of their uterus. Here there are no stitches. In most cases, the kidney will soon start producing urine.

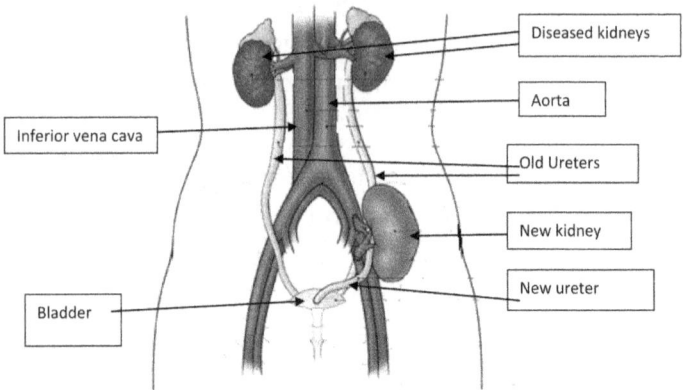

Depending on its quality, the new kidney usually begins functioning immediately. Living donor kidneys normally require 3–5 days to reach normal functioning levels, while cadaveric donations stretch that interval to 7–15 days. Hospital stay is typically for 4–7 days.

Immunosuppressant drugs are used to suppress the immune system from rejecting the donor kidney. These medicines must be taken for the rest of the recipient's life.

Normally HLA and ABO matching are done between donor and recipient, so that there is no rejection of the kidney. But after availability of powerful and effective immune suppressive drugs, even an un-related, genetically different donor can donate the kidney.

Contraindications to transplantation — if a person has any of these problems, he cannot undergo transplantation

- Heart failure
- Respiratory failure

- Liver failure

- Severe obesity

- Severe infection

- Cancer

- Severe mental problems

- Tobacco, alcohol and drug addicts

- Any other reason where the patient cannot be subjected to major surgery

Paid donor transplant is illegal in India, but legal in Iran, Australia and Singapore. Actually the cost comes down when it is legal, since price can be standardized. There is also less chance of exploitation of the poor who donate a kidney to earn some money.

Kidney Pancreas transplant

In a Diabetic with renal failure, it makes sense to transplant Kidneys and Pancreas at the same time especially in Type-1 Diabetes. Or only some islet cells (that secrete insulin) from a living/dead donor can be performed, either with or after kidney transplant. This involves taking a deceased donor pancreas, breaking it down, and extracting the Islet cells that make insulin. The cells are then injected through a catheter into the recipient and they generally lodge in the liver. The recipient still needs to take drugs to avoid rejection, but no surgery is required. Most people need two or three such injections; many are not completely insulin-free although their doses come down.

Transplant patients are supposed to avoid grapefruit, green tea and pomegranate because they interfere with transplant medication

Rejection of the transplanted kidney occurs in 10–25% of people after transplant during the first 60 days. Rejection does not necessarily mean loss of the organ, but it may necessitate additional medication.

The average lifetime for a donated kidney is ten to fifteen years. When a transplant fails, a patient may opt for a second transplant, and may have to return to dialysis for some intermediary time.

- Bill Thompson is the longest-surviving American kidney recipient from an unrelated donor, having received his kidney in 1966 at age 15; it has survived over 40 years.

- Chakravarthy from Chennai, India, received kidney from his brother on 2 May 1983 at the age of 29, is still alive and healthy 27 years later.

CHAPTER 17

DIABETES IN PREGNANCY – GDM (GESTATIONAL DIABETES MELLITUS)

Gestational Diabetes is a condition in which pregnant women who are not previously diabetic, exhibit high blood glucose levels—"any degree of glucose intolerance with onset or first recognition during pregnancy". This is seen especially during the third trimester (after 6 months) and in 3-10% of population.

Risk factors for GDM

- Polycystic Ovary Syndrome. Ovaries are the egg producing organs in the female body that lie on either side of the uterus or womb. They are responsible for formation of eggs which are then implanted in the uterus for fertilization with the sperm. When there is hormonal imbalance, small sacs or cysts develop in them. This leads to interference in their functioning, and further hormonal imbalance. There is increase in weight, growth of hair over body, menstrual irregularity, and even development of Diabetes

UTERUS – front view

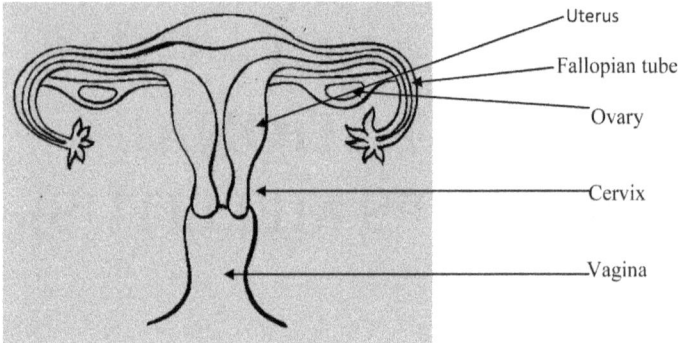

Now who is likely to get GDM? —

- A previous diagnosis of gestational diabetes or prediabetes, impaired glucose tolerance.

- A family history revealing a first-degree relative with type 2 diabetes

- Maternal age - a woman's risk factor increases as she gets older (especially for women over 35 years of age).

- Minority groups (those with higher risk factors include African-Americans, Afro-Caribbeans, Native Americans, Hispanics, Pacific Islanders, and people originating from South East Asia)

- Smoking — doubles the risk

- Being overweight, obese or severely obese increases the risk –BMI over 30kg/sq M

- A previous pregnancy which resulted in a child with a big baby (high birth weight: >4 kg (8 lbs)

- Previous difficulty in labour

- Other genetic risk factors: There are at least 10 genes that are associated with an increased risk of gestational diabetes.

Diagnosis of GDM

GDM is ideally diagnosed by OGTT (oral glucose tolerance test). It should be performed in the morning after an overnight fast of between 8 and 14 hours. During the three previous days the subject must have an unrestricted diet (containing at least 150 g carbohydrate per day) and unlimited physical activity. The subject should remain seated and not smoke throughout the test.

The test involves drinking a solution containing a certain amount of glucose, usually 75 g or 100 g, and drawing blood to measure glucose levels at the start and set time intervals.

100 gms OGTT will detect more cases than the 75gms OGTT. But some pregnant women cannot tolerate so much glucose and tend to have nausea (vomiting sensation) because of it. In these people 'a non challenge glucose test' can be done. Here glucose is not given but simple fasting and two hour post meal test is performed.

All high risk cases should be screened for GDM. But 40-60% of patients do not have any risk factor but develop GDM. Therefore ideally all women should be screened when first detected to be pregnant and again around 24-28 weeks.

Criteria for diagnosis of gestational diabetes according to Indian National Diabetes Data group after 75 grams glucose –

- Fasting – below105 mg/dl
- 1 hour - below 190 mg/dl
- 2 hours - below165 mg/dl
- 3 hour - below145 mg/dl

Criteria for diagnosis of GDM with non-challenge blood glucose test (no glucose).

This is performed by taking fasting and two hours after a meal, similar to diagnosis of Diabetes in a non pregnant lady.

When a plasma glucose level is found to be higher than 126 mg/dl after fasting, or over 200 mg/dl post meal, and if this is confirmed on a subsequent day, the diagnosis of GDM is made.

Complaints

Typically, women with GDM exhibit no symptoms (another reason for universal screening), but some women may demonstrate increased thirst, increased urination, fatigue, nausea, vomiting, fungal infections, and blurred vision.

Why GDM occurs

During pregnancy, several hormones are secreted in high amounts—like cortisol, prolactin, oestrogen, progesterone. All these hormones, increase blood sugar. To counteract their effect, more insulin is secreted. But in some ladies, this increased secretion of insulin may not be enough, resulting in high blood sugar, and Diabetes.

Management

Diet should be high calorie (to provide enough nutrition for pregnancy), but simple carbohydrates should be excluded. Complex carbohydrates with a lowGI(see GI tables—in chapter on Diet) should be advised and spread through the day. Simple carbohydrates should especially be avoided in the morning since insulin resistance is highest at that time. Carbohydrates from whole grains, fruits and vegetables are best.

Regular moderately intense physical exercise is advised.

Regular blood check up for blood sugar and HbA1c are also advised

If a diabetic diet or G.I. Diet, exercise, and oral medication are inadequate to control glucose levels, insulin therapy may become necessary.

A repeat OGTT should be carried out 6 weeks after delivery, to confirm the diabetes has disappeared. Afterwards, regular screening for type 2 diabetes is advised.

Chances of getting Diabetes in future

- Gestational diabetes generally resolves once the baby is born. Based on different studies, the chances of developing GDM in a second pregnancy, if you had GDM in your first pregnancy, are between 30 and 84%. The risk is highest in women who needed insulin treatment.

The following carry a higher risk —

- A second pregnancy within 1 year of the previous pregnancy
- Multiple pregnancies
- Those that needed insulin
- Those with glutamate decarboxylase, antibodies or insulinoma antigen-2
- The risk appears to be highest in the first 5 years
- 50-70% after 11 years
- 25% after 15 years

COMPLICATIONS OF GDM

Complications in mother

- Birth trauma as babies are big
- swelling, raised blood pressure, chances of fits
- Forceps and other assisted delivery
- Increased incidence of cesarean section
- Long-term risk of developing diabetes

- Metabolic syndrome — Diabetes, Hypertension and ,raised lipids

Complications in baby

- large baby
- low sugar in the new born for about a week after birth
- liver involvement
- increased risk of death around birth
- birth defects
- increase in red cells
- low calcium, magnesium
- Respiratory distress syndrome — severe breathing disease
- Birth trauma — injury to shoulder, fracture collar bone, paralysis of 5th -7th nerves in neck.

Complications in child later in life

- Obesity
- Diabetes

PREVENTION OF GDM

GDM may be prevented by taking care of risk factors, especially — PCOD, stoppage of smoking, regular exercise, and weight reduction. At least it may not manifest in a very severe form even in the high risk cases.

PART IV

Prevention and reversal of Diabetes

CHAPTER 18

Prevention of diabetes

Ha Ha!

Eat right, reduce weight, exercise more or alter your genetic code to prevent Diabetes!

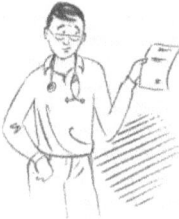

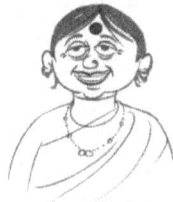

Can diabetes be prevented? Type -1 Diabetes that has a very strong genetic basis cannot be prevented, but it can be postponed.

Type-2 that begins later in life can be prevented although it too has a genetic basis — by keeping weight in check, exercising regularly, and starting a diabetic diet if there is a very strong family history.

Insulin resistance

Since this is the basic cause of Type-2 Diabetes, detecting and correcting it can help in preventing Diabetes. How can we diagnose insulin resistance? — We can perform tests like -QUICKI, HOMA, insulin tolerance tests, insulin levels in blood, insulin suppression tests etc discussed already.

So those of you with a strong family history consult your doctor and undergo these tests to detect insulin resistance early and try to correct it — thus preventing Diabetes.

CHAPTER 19

CAN DIABETES BE REVERSED?

Now we are going to address this very fascinating topic — reversal of Diabetes

What is reversal?

Diabetes has always been considered incurable, and a lifelong problem once diagnosed. Then how are we suddenly talking about its reversal? Are we speaking about some new kind of fad treatment that has suddenly been discovered? No! Let me caution you — *by reversal I do not mean cure.* Reversal means trying to go backwards instead of forward. If you are on a certain dose of insulin, you can try to reduce it and if possible, stop it altogether and go on oral tablets. If you are on a heavy dose of oral medication, you can try to reduce it to a minimal number and if possible even stop all medication. But reversal does not mean that you become totally free of Diabetes lifelong. You have to continue to monitor and stick to the lifestyle changes that helped you reverse your Diabetes. Once that is understood, let us proceed further.

Let me tell you how this thought process of trying to reverse Diabetes started —

In the last decade or so, Bariatric surgery for obesity, has become very common. And in many patients after Bariatric surgery, it was found that their blood glucose came to normal as early as within three days after surgery which had nothing to do with weight loss. In fact MRI performed within a few weeks of surgery, showed a rapid reduction in liver fat and improvement in insulin sensitivity, followed by reduction in pancreatic fat deposition and return of normal functioning of Pancreas. As we have understood earlier, *these are the changes that lead to Diabetes*. So it got doctors thinking — how did this reversal happen?

Actually they deduced it is the *sudden and very drastic reduction in calories* that led to these positive changes; since in bariatric surgery, you reduce the size of the stomach you can only eat so much. Now, doctors pondered — could a low calorie diet work the same way as Bariatric surgery in reversing Diabetes?

We know that insulin secreted by Pancreas suppresses glucose output from liver. But fat inside the liver prevents this action of insulin and glucose continues to be released from liver into the blood . In addition, excess fat from the liver spills over into the blood as fatty acids and is deposited in the Pancreas. Here it prevents insulin release after meals. Excessive fat in the Pancreas also leads to death of Beta cells that release insulin. *So Diabetes is actually a disease of too much fat inside the organs.*

Excess of carbohydrates are also converted into fat and stored in the body if they remain unutilized for energy. Actually refined carbohydrates are a bigger culprit than fat in the diet. If we consume more fat, it can be deposited in liver, under the skin or in other organs. But consuming too much of refined carbohydrates leads to their conversion into fat *that is stored only in liver.*

Bariatric surgery and reversal of Diabetes — experience worldwide

In Bariatric surgery, the size of the stomach is reduced either by banding, cutting off a 'sleeve' from the stomach or 'by passing' it.

Roux – en – Y Gastric Bypass

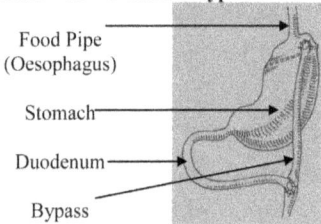

Food Pipe (Oesophagus)

Stomach

Duodenum

Bypass

Banded Gastroplasty

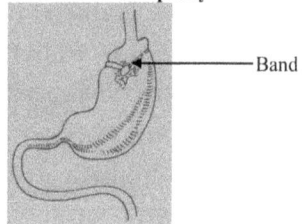

Band

Sleeve gastrectomy

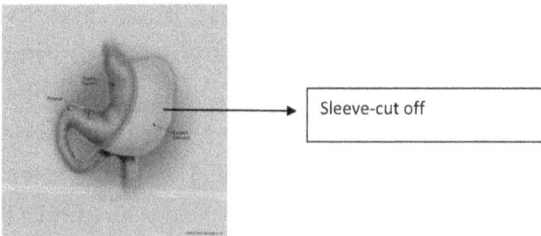

Sleeve-cut off

This results in a sudden and drastic reduction in calorie intake resulting in reversal of Diabetes as we have already discussed. The 'by-pass' procedure shows the best results. So there seems to be a mechanism beyond caloric restriction. Are there any risks of Bariatric surgery? Immediate risk is small — 0.3% chance of death within 30 days. But there can be infection leaking from stomach into the abdominal cavity, gallstones because of accumulation of extra fat released from liver and nutritional deficiency leading to conditions like thinning and weakness of bones and anaemia.

A 2008 study of 55 obese patients found that 73 percent of those who underwent gastric banding saw their diabetes disappear after two years, compared to 13 percent undergoing standard medical treatment such as medication, diet and exercise. Gastric banding has of course now almost become obsolete because of the superiority of the other methods of bariatric surgery.

In 2009, surgeons at the University of Minnesota analyzed 621 mostly small studies of bariatric surgery in obese, diabetic patients. Their conclusion, reported in the American Journal of Medicine: 78 percent no longer needed medication to control their blood sugar. Their Diabetes had been reversed. But most patients in these studies were obese, many morbidly so. (The average BMI was 48.) The improvement in glucose control could therefore be credited to the patients' weight loss, which averaged 85 pounds. But in many patients the blood glucose normalised within days, much before weight reduction happened.

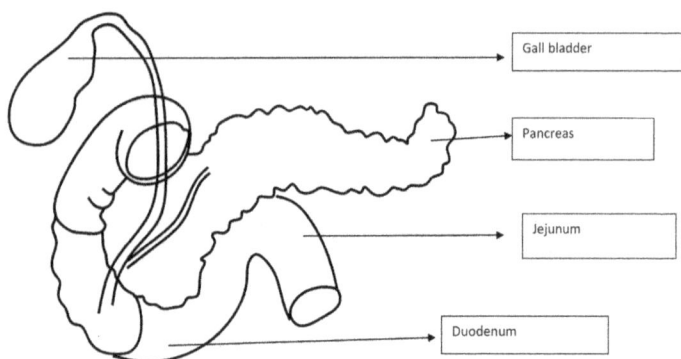

Now, some reseachers tried connecting the stomach directly to the second part of the intestines called jejunum They called this DJB or duodeno-jejunal-bypass. Curiously, although patients shed a few pounds, there was no correlation between weight loss and blood glucose. They propounded this theory — normally, the jejunum receives well digested mush. But after DJB it directly receives undigested food from the stomach since duodenum has been bypassed. And it sends a signal to the brain — 'got glucose! 'Brain thinks there is abundance of glucose, so it sends a signal to liver — 'stop production of glucose!' and blood glucose comes down, leading to reversal of Diabetes

But gastric surgery for Diabetes should be reserved for obese patients who have failed to manage their disease with more conventional interventions, such as diet, exercise and medications since any surgery can potentially have complications.

In one study, most surgery patients were able to stop all diabetes drugs and have their disease stay in remission for at least two years.

Ileal transposition and reversal

This is another surgery, where the end of the intestines called ileum is brought up and connected to the second part of the intestines called jejunum. There is secretion of a chemical called 'incretin' from the ileum, which causes release of insulin from Pancreas. Since ileum has been brought closer to Pancreas, incretin from it acts more efficiently — increasing insulin secretion after food intake, and thereby lowering blood glucose.

Is reversal possible without surgery?

To mimic Bariatric surgery, doctors advised a low calorie diet consisting of 600 kcals from a totally fat free diet, with complex carbohydrates and non-fat proteins for 8 weeks. Three liters of water or non fizzy, non sweetened simple fluids to assuage hunger pangs, and 200 calories from vegetables –simply cooked or in salad form. Along with diet, large muscle exercise with weights and bands — to help in uptake of glucose by muscles, was also advised.

With this diet, an average loss of weight was 15.3 kg over the 8-week period. This is similar to weight loss after gastric bypass. The liver had normalized in the group with diabetes. Liver fat fell by 30% during the first 7 days of negative energy balance. This reduction in liver fat improved insulin sensitivity in the liver and reduced production of glucose by it. Insulin response to food also increased so that, after 8 weeks of diet, it had increased to within the normal range. The B-cells had woken up! This had never been demonstrated before. And since effective insulin was available, there was no need to keep secreting excessive insulin as used to happen earlier. Clearly, the B-cells are not permanently damaged in Type 2 diabetes, but are merely suppressed. Now the question—Is long-standing Type 2 diabetes reversible? We now know of many people reversing long duration Type 2 diabetes (one person after 28 years) following either a hypo caloric diet or bariatric surgery.

Let us go back and remember in reverse as to how Diabetes occurs. *chronic and sustained high calorie diet leads to fat accumulation in liver in people who have Diabetic genes.* The story begins with resistance to action of insulin in muscles. This leads to high insulin levels in blood, which in turn leads to fat deposition in liver. So a low calorie diet – *(only 25% of normal calories are given for eight weeks)* achieved dramatic results. Not only was there a rapid fall in blood glucose, fat content of Pancreas and liver came down dramatically, with a weight reduction of about 15 kg which was comparable to Bariatric surgery without the side effects of the latter. During severe calorie reduction, the person can feel weak and giddy, *but as long as he can sustain, he must continue.* Later, calorie reduction of lesser intensity, changing quality of food, and regular exercise can maintain the reversal. *Once the basic cause – that is fat accumulation in liver and pancreas is removed, these organs start functioning properly again and Diabetes can be reversed.*

Is it easy?—NO! But any patient with courage and a strong will power can try it. If not complete reversal, at least a drastic reduction in medication will *definitely be achieved and further progress checked*. That in itself will be a huge achievement. Continuous motivation and family support will help in achieving good results.

Is a slow reversal possible?

Many of you will not be able to manage a drastic caloric reduction and sustain it for 8 weeks. For you, a slow reversal can be tried. Let me now give you an example of one of my patients — let us call her XY. She had been suffering from Diabetes for the past 8 years and was on 6 tablets a day of oral medication and 7 kg overweight as per ideal body weight requirements for her height. I put her on a complex carbohydrate, low fat, adequate protein, adequate fibre diet

There was no calorie counting but she was made to understand the principles of her diet. Salads, sprouts, cooked vegetables and fruits were to be evenly distributed throughout the day and the rest of the food eaten as desired.

She was also asked to climb a hill 2000 ft high near her home everyday — spending at least an hour. Committed person that she was, XY did that twice a day. She also tested and monitored her blood sugar so often, that she says her finger tips were like pin cushions.

In six months she had lost the extra 7 kg weight she was carrying, BMI came down from 25 to 22, waist circumference came down from 86cm to 83 cm, her biological age was 63 but metabolic age now showed 43 years. Her HbA1c has remained under 7% in spite of taking only a third of the medication she was on 6 months back. She is now fitter, slimmer, and more importantly from 6 tablets a day, she is down to 1, and the improvement is continuing. Of course there are temporary setbacks, but she claws her way back.

She is now highly motivated to bring down her HbA1c below 6.4% (pre Diabetes) and then below 5.7%.(non Diabetic) range, and then stop all medication. *So, slow reversal is also possible in a highly motivated person.* Also, once the fat disappears from liver, Pancreas, omentum, and your(BMR) basic metabolic rate goes up, and your muscles start using glucose, the reversal process continues. Even if she does not achieve complete reversal, she has achieved quite a bit don't you think?

Precautions during attempted reversal

- Drugs that act by secreting insulin can be stopped totally. Insulin can be gradually reduced by monitoring sugar regularly; other medicines like 'metformin' can be gradually reduced.

- Usually a 15 kg weight loss in 8 weeks is desirable to reverse Diabetes. Those who are only slightly overweight can try to achieve a BMI that is just below normal.

- If a patient has moderate or severe retinopathy(eye involvement), he should be screened after six months of beginning the attempt at reversal, since the sudden reduction in retinal blood flow associated with the return of normal blood glucose control can be bad for areas of the retina with reduced circulation resulting possibly in worsening of retinopathy

For those individuals who achieve reversal of their type 2 diabetes, retinal screening should be continued for two years if there is no pre-existing retinopathy.

If retinopathy is present, it should be continued until all changes come to normal.

All major complications will improve with the dietary changes. It should be noted that blood pressure control will be substantially improved, with the possibility of decreasing number or dose of anti-hypertensive agents.

In fact weight reduction alone can reverse many diseases like Hypertension, Diabetes, Thyroid deficiency, lipid disorders; and prevent ischaemic heart disease, arthritis, back problems, cancer, varicose veins, and many others. So most important treatment for Diabetes is to bring down body weight 10% below your normal desired weight. It might be bit difficult for you in the beginning but as you see the results, you will be strongly motivated. Remember —

" Today it hurts , tomorrow it works "

Is diabetes with normal BMI reversible?

Yes: even a person of Type 2 Diabetes with normal BMI has fat accumulation in liver that can be corrected by a low calorie diet for 8 weeks. Any severe weight loss should later be re-gained in the form of increase in muscle mass with exercise.

Final verdict

So what's the final verdict? Is reversal possible? Yes I think so. Definitely with Bariatric surgery; *but in a committed person, it is possible without surgery.* Many studies have indicated that Diabetes can be reversed with calorie restriction — as little as 600 kcal a day for a 8 week period; and losing up to 15kg weight, as long as there are still some functioning B-cells in the Pancreas to secrete insulin. An MRI can reveal to what degree your Pancreatic cells have been destroyed.

And you can also attempt a slower reversal as in the case of my patient-XY.

The trick is in eating low glycaemic foods, every few hours in small quantities and monitoring and adjusting doses of drugs frequently. Mindful eating is essential. Eat slowly, chew thoroughly as our grandmothers advised over twenty minutes. It will satisfy 'satiety or fullness centre' in the brain with less food

And like I said earlier, *the worst case scenario will be a drastic reduction in dosage of medicine*. That in itself for most of you will be a huge achievement. So go for it!

There is another patient of mine who has reversed his Diabetes. He has come down from 68.5 kg in 2004 when he was first detected with Diabetes to 53 kg in 11 years. In January 2015 he suffered a heart attack and went on such a strict diet and life style modification that he lost 7-8 kg very rapidly — this led to the reversal and it is maintained even now after 11 months in December 2015. Since he is underweight, I am now trying to get him to bulk up his muscles.

There are many other patients of mine who have reversed their Diabetes to a great degree.

CHAPTER 20

Targets, summary of guidelines and common queries

Here are a few common queries—

Why did I get it?

Many people, who get Diabetes, are overweight, do not exercise, and have no control over their diet. But there are others who lead a disciplined life and have normal weight, and still get Diabetes. These patients want to know why they got Diabetes.

In such patients there is a strong genetic basis; and it surfaces whenever there is a stressful condition like a severe infection or illness, or an emotional crisis. During these conditions, there is increased demand for insulin that cannot be met and Diabetes results. Many of these patients may be able to tide over this episode, and manage their Diabetes with lifestyle changes. But sometime or the other, full- fledged Diabetes is bound to occur. Only a few who never relax their lifestyle remain free of overt Diabetes, lifelong.

Can a thin person get Diabetes?

Sure, if there is a strong genetic basis – he can. Many people are thin but are 'apple shaped' – with more belly girth – see picture below that you have seen previously. These people have fat stored between and in their organs in the abdomen called visceral fat and are more likely to get Diabetes. Conversely, there are many fat people who are 'pear shaped' with more fat around their hips. These people rarely get Diabetes. So if a thin person has the genes, he *can* get Diabetes.

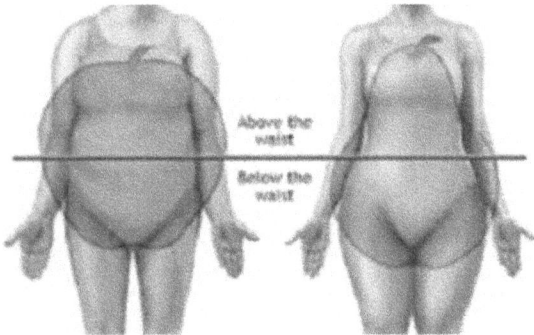

I have a strong genetic history, can I avoid getting Diabetes?

Sure! If you keep your BMI and waist circumference normal, eat right, exercise regularly and avoid stress, you can avoid getting Diabetes.

If I am able to reverse my Diabetes, will it be permanent?

No – you will have to continue with intensive Life style changes of diet and exercise and avoid re-accumulation of fat in organs to maintain the reversal.

TARGETS FOR CARDIAC AND DIABETIC PATIENTS

BMI	≤23Kg/m2
BP	≤130/80
FBS	≤100mg%
PPBS	≤140mg%
HbA1C	≤7%
CHOLESTEROL	≤150mg%
TRIGLYCERIDES	≤150mg%
HDL	≥45mg%
LDL	≤70mg%
B-12	≥250pg/ml
D-3	≥30ng/ml
URINE MICRAL	≤20mg%
URINE ALB/CREAT RATIO	≤30mcg/mg

Summary of guidelines for Diabetics

- Strictly follow prescribed diet
- Never miss a meal
- Reduce your weight
- Get adequate sleep
- Do not change dose of medication without consulting your doctor
- Always carry some sweets with you in case your blood sugar goes down
- Exercise regularly

- Test urine & blood sugar regularly

- Stop smoking

- Avoid exposure to infections

- Attend immediately to wounds on any part of body

- Always wear comfortable footwear & loose cotton clothing

- Non-nutritive sweeteners are safe when consumed within the acceptable daily intake levels.

- Limit alcohol intake to a moderate amount (one drink per day).

- Routine supplementation with antioxidants or chromium supplementation is not advised.

- Carry a diabetic card

- Take care of any foot infection under the guidance of your doctor, with proper antibiotics, local cleaning, dressing, and rest, to avoid weight bearing on the limb, till healing occurs.

- Avoid self pity and see how you can improve control.

- Keep in regular touch with your physician, as newer & better drugs are constantly coming into the market

- Be positive and unstressed.

  And you can change —

From this —

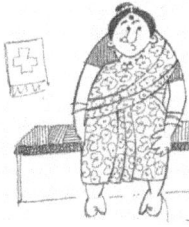

From this

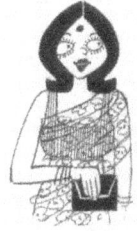

to this

CONCLUSION

The purpose of this book was to equip the reader with enough theoretical and practical knowledge to be able to manage 60% of his Diabetes on his own — this can be acheived with proper understanding of his disease, including diet, exercise, reducing weight, body care, recognizing and knowing how to prevent complications, self-monitoring etc — which I hope has been achieved. Once that was done, an attempt at reversal could be tried.

Diabetes is a chronic and complex disease that can be difficult to manage. But you will find that once you understand your disease fully and *participate* in its management things will become easier. When you are told 'do this/don't do this!' by your doctor, it seems as if the responsibility of managing your problem rests fully with him; and you continue to play a secondary role. You go for your appointment once in three months, but may remain immune to any amount of counseling or attempt to scare you with threats of complications. Only a few fully motivated patients are completely compliant. But once you are aware that not only are you going to participate in the management of your disease, but that *you* are going to be the *major partner*, you will be more responsible and try to fully understand every aspect of Diabetes. Now magically you will find that results will improve. There is almost going to be a role reversal. Instead of saying 'do this/ don't do this!' your doctor may ask 'so what have you achieved this time?' After all, you have been fully trained in self-management, and results are expected from you!

This is also the time to awaken the competitive spirit in you. You can form something like a 'towel club' with other Diabetic patients known to you; where everyone comes with a towel, pours out their problems and cries into their towel. After some time, you will all realize that others' problems are equal or more severe than yours and slowly you throw away the towel to become more positive about your disease. You compare results — sugar, HbA1c, weight, and all the parameters you have been taught to track and rejoice at each other's success. Now everyone is happy — you, your doctor, and those close to you. In fact it is a good idea to involve at least one member of the family. And if your spouse is also a diabetic, it becomes easier. I want to give you a few more hints in self-management —

Never be ashamed of declaring that you are a diabetic. This is one of the common reasons for poor control. You go to a party or to someone's house, and since you have not told them you are a diabetic; they offer you sweets, which you accept thinking — once in a while it doesn't matter. But believe me it keeps adding up!

Let there be no excuses for avoiding exercise — rain, sunshine, cold, fog, guests, or functions — stick to your exercise routine. After all you never stop eating do you?

Reward yourself once in a while with safe sweet alternatives or a deep fried item if *you* feel you've earned it.

Good control means **monitoring**; the more frequently you monitor the more chances of better control.

Good control also means maintain **regularity** in your lifestyle.

There will be umpteen number of people telling you about umpteen alternate therapies that can 'cure' your Diabetes. You can try them out under your doctor's supervision, but please continue your regular medication and monitoring. I am not saying all of them are useless. But I have many cases where patients have stopped their regular medication after starting these alternate therapies — with disastrous consequences.

Like I've said before, there are bound to be setbacks, and you have to be prepared to take them in your stride and move on. A lot of what I have said in this book might have scared you. But believe me it is intentional — I do *want* to scare you. Once you have Diabetes, you should have FEAR that you may develop its dreaded complications But FEAR should not be 'Forget Everything and Run away' — remember *you can't run away* , FEAR should be 'Face Everything And Rise' or 'Face everything and reverse'!

But I certainly do not want you to be unhappy either. Learn to live with Diabetes with intense involvement, while living your life as happily as you can. Actually you will find it's not that bad. Once you get into a regular routine, you will start enjoying it.

Remember—Normal sugar=Normal life expectancy!

With proper care and a positive attitude, diabetics can enjoy a normal span of life. And if you are prepared to work hard, you can even reverse your Diabetes. And hopefully in the near future, we will have a permanent cure for diabetes. Let that sweet thought sustain you!

And—here is a poem I wrote to motivate you!

Diabetes is a difficult disease it is true

It affects all ages and of every hue

turning your body black and blue

And lasts your whole life too

Quite unlike the common flu —

You can't kick it away it is true

So you got to remember the don'ts and the do's

And the instructions that are hardly a few

But —

Fight it, tide it, ride it and see it through

since advanced treatments emerging from the blue

for its cure are giving doctors a clue —

To charge you up all anew!

ABOUT THE AUTHOR

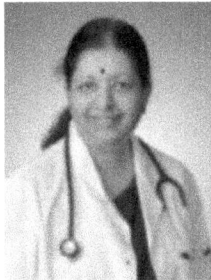

DR. GEETA SUNDAR M.D
Medical consultant, Diabetologist and author

I did my Indian school certificate (formerly senior Cambridge) from St. Joseph's convent Jabalpur with merit in English literature. I was always interested in writing, and won several prizes for essay and prose both in school and college. Later I joined MBBS and went on to do my post graduation in medicine. Passed WHO recognised certificate course in Diabetes. I have been practicing as a consultant in medicine for more than 30 years, and as Diabetologist for five years. In 2002 I started writing, first health books and then fiction.

Other activities

Regular contributor to Times wellness

Chief medical advisor to 'India online health'

Corporate lecturer

CONTACT

healthauthorpune@gmail.com

sundar.geeta@gmail.com

PICTURES OF MY EIGHT BOOKS

1) The Premier Murder League–Penguin —a T-20 murder mystery

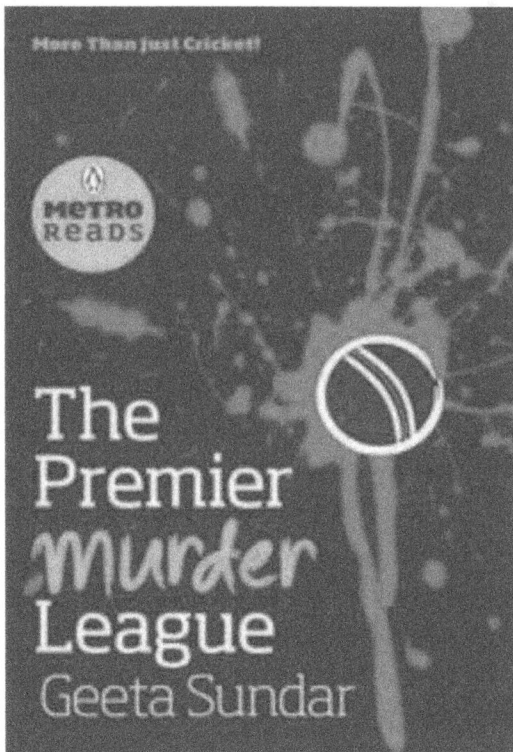

From Macmillan web-site (both my books have been declared best sellers)

2) Health after Forty

Health After Forty Best seller

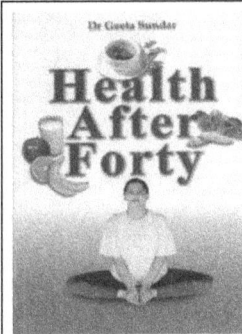

Author(s)	:	Geeta Sundar
ISBN	:	9780333938959
Imprint	:	M a c m i l l a n P u b l i s h e r s India
Copyright	:	2002
Trim Size	:	5.5" x 8.5"
Pages	:	260
Binding	:	Paperback
List Price	:	Rs. 210.00
Language	:	English

About the Book

This book equips readers with the knowledge to combat health problems that arise after the age of forty and explains how this change brings with it physical disturbances and mental discontent. Common ailments that often afflict people are identified and possible preventives and remedies are suggested. The author also suggests lifestyle and dietary modifications that are necessary to equip a person to deal with post-forty afflictions.

3) A-Z of Bone Muscle and joint diseases

A to Z of Bones Muscles and Joint Diseases : A Practical

Guide to Become a Well Informed Patient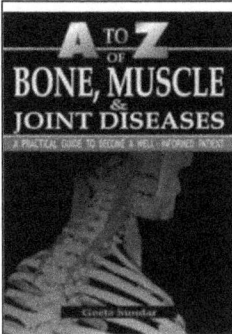

Author(s)	:	Dr Geeta Sundar
ISBN	:	9781403926708
Imprint	:	M a c m i l l a n Publishers India
Copyright	:	2005
Trim Size	:	5.5″ x 8.5″
Pages	:	192
Binding	:	Paperback
List Price	:	Rs. 185.00
Language	:	English

4) Sterling Publishers–Contributor

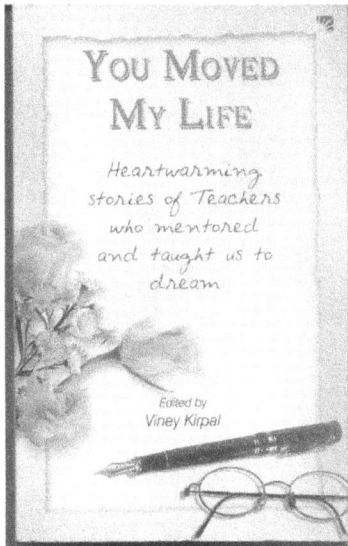

5) Macmillan

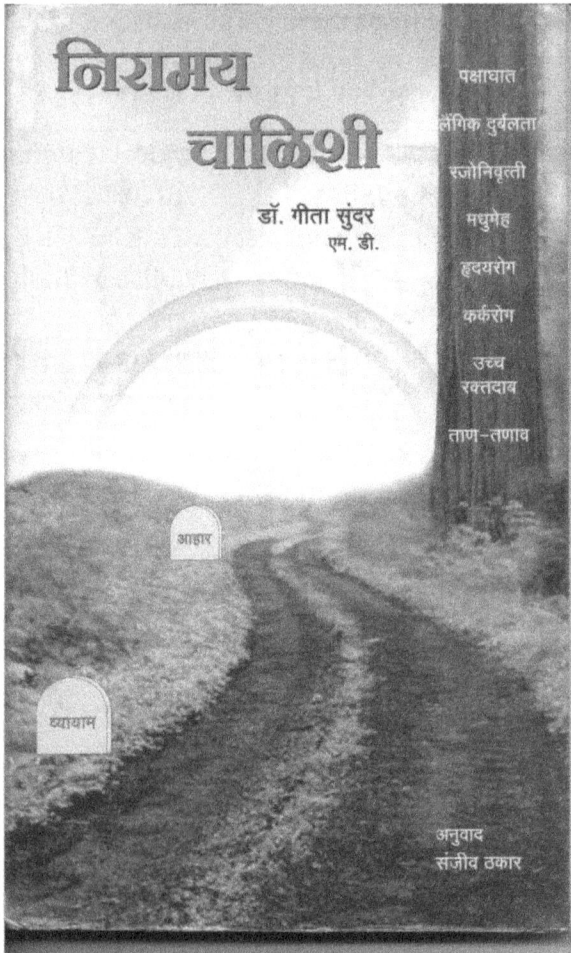

निरामय
चालिशी

डॉ. गीता सुंदर
एम. डी.

पक्षाघात
लैंगिक दुर्बलता
रजोनिवृत्ती
मधुमेह
हृदयरोग
कर्करोग
उच्च
रक्तदाब
ताण-तणाव

आहार

व्यायाम

अनुवाद
संजीव ठकार

6) Amazon—'Constipation can be managed safely'

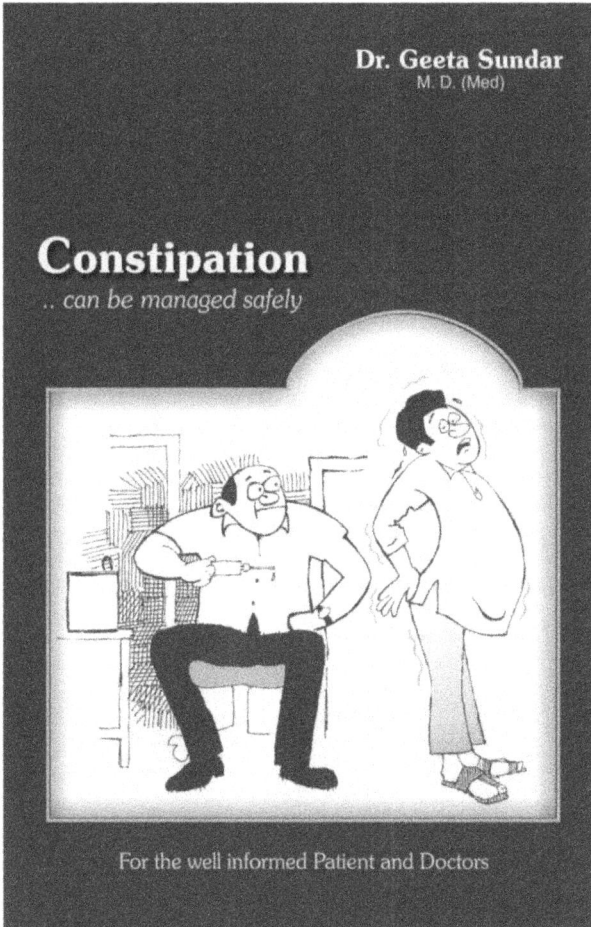

7) Smile a while doc — self published

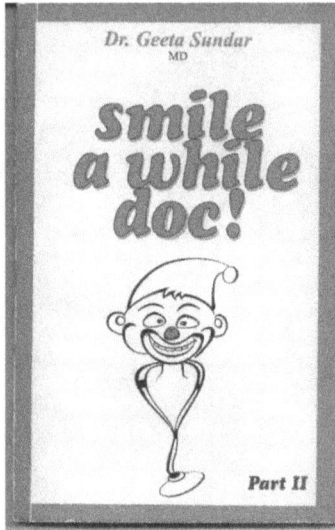

8) She writes — Random house — twelve prize winning authors

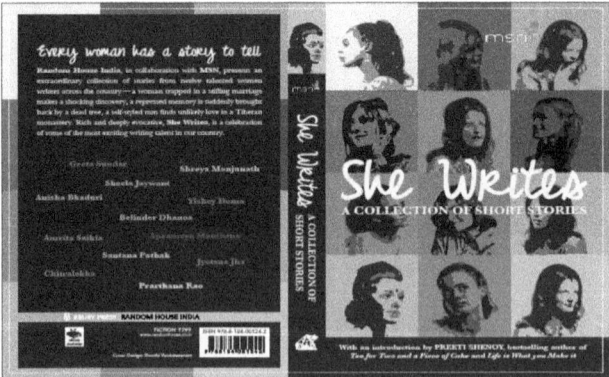